The Dream Body Blueprint: Building Your Dream Physique

Bogdan Pashchynskiy

Published by Bogdan Pashchynskiy, 2023.

THE DREAM BODY BLUEPRINT: BUILDING YOUR DREAM PHYSIQUE

ISBN: 978-91-527-7324-6

Written by Bogdan Pashchynskiy.

Table of Contents

I: Introduction
Why This Book Was Made

This book was created with a clear purpose: to empower and guide individuals on their fitness journey toward achieving their goals and transforming their bodies. It was crafted with a deep understanding of the challenges and obstacles that many face when navigating the complex world of fitness, nutrition, and mindset.

The motivation behind this book stems from the belief that everyone deserves the opportunity to unlock their full potential and create the body and lifestyle they desire. It was made to provide a comprehensive resource that combines scientific knowledge, practical strategies, and actionable advice to help readers take control of their fitness, make informed choices, and achieve sustainable results.

Through the pages of this book, you will find a wealth of information, insights, and practical tools that have been carefully curated to support you on your journey. Whether you are a beginner looking to kickstart your fitness routine, an experienced individual seeking to break through plateaus, or someone wanting to optimize their health and well-being, this book has something for you.

We understand that embarking on a fitness transformation is not always easy. It requires dedication, perseverance, and a solid understanding of the principles that drive progress. That's why this book goes beyond surface-level advice and dives deep into the science and psychology behind effective training, nutrition, and mindset strategies.

Our goal is to provide you with the knowledge and tools you need to make informed decisions, set realistic goals, and develop a sustainable approach to your fitness journey. We want to equip you with the understanding to navigate through the noise of conflicting information and fad diets and instead empower you to make choices that align with your unique needs and aspirations.

Remember, this book is not just about physical transformations; it's about personal growth and self-discovery. It's about developing a positive mindset, building resilience, and embracing the journey towards your goals. We encourage you to approach this book with an open mind, ready to absorb the knowledge and insights shared within its pages.

Ultimately, this book was made for you—for your success, your well-being, and your transformation. We hope that it serves as a trusted companion on your path to a stronger, healthier, and more fulfilling life.

Let's embark on this journey together!

The Benefits of Having a Fit and Healthy Body

Having a healthy and fit body brings a multitude of benefits that extend far beyond physical appearance. It's not just about looking good; it's about feeling good and living a fulfilling life. Here are some key benefits that await those who commit to prioritizing their health and fitness:

1. Enhanced Energy and Vitality: A healthy and fit body translates into boundless energy and vitality that infuses every aspect of your life. You'll find yourself waking up with enthusiasm, tackling challenges with vigor, and embracing each day with a renewed zest for life. With increased energy levels, you'll have the capacity to accomplish more and fully enjoy all that life has to offer.

2. Improved Physical Health: Regular exercise and proper nutrition contribute to a stronger immune system, improved cardiovascular health, and reduced risk of chronic diseases. Your body becomes more resilient, and you're better equipped to ward off illnesses, recover faster from ailments, and maintain optimal physical well-being. A healthy body empowers you to live life to the fullest, free from the burdens of preventable health issues.

3. Mental Clarity and Focus: Physical fitness has a profound impact on mental clarity and cognitive function. Engaging in regular exercise releases endorphins, the "feel-good" hormones, which help alleviate stress, boost mood and enhance mental well-being. A fit body promotes mental clarity, sharpens focus, and improves overall cognitive performance, enabling you to excel in various areas of life, whether it's work, studies, or personal pursuits.

4. Increased Confidence and Self-Esteem: Achieving and maintaining a healthy body nurtures a sense of accomplishment and boosts self-confidence. As you witness your progress, whether it's reaching fitness milestones, shedding excess weight, or gaining strength, your confidence grows. Feeling good in your own skin radiates positive energy, and it positively impacts your interactions with others. Confidence and self-esteem become your companions, empowering you to pursue your dreams and face life's challenges head-on.

5. Stress Relief and Emotional Well-being: Exercise is a powerful stress reliever and mood enhancer. Engaging in physical activity helps release tension, reduce anxiety, and alleviate symptoms of depression. It provides an outlet for emotional expression, clearing the mind and bringing a sense of peace and balance. A healthy body becomes a sanctuary, allowing you to cope with the demands of daily life more effectively and cultivate emotional well-being.

These are just a few of the many benefits that a healthy and fit body can bring to your life. By beginning this journey, you are investing in your long-term well-being and setting the stage for a vibrant, fulfilling, and empowered existence. So, let's discover the incredible potential that lies within you.

14 Things This Book Will Help You Achieve

Build a strong and fit body.

Gain muscle mass.

Look physically appealing and aesthetic.

Lose fat sustainably and effectively.

Improve your cardiovascular fitness and endurance.

Optimize your nutrition and create meal plans.

Enhance flexibility and mobility.

Become more disciplined, increase motivation, and improve your mindset.

Enhance your sleep and recovery.

Optimize your hormone levels.

Improve your mental well-being.

Prevent and manage injuries.

Set goals and track progress.

Bust fitness myths.

Nine Suggestions On How To Get The Most Out Of This Book

1. To truly maximize the value of this book, there is one essential requirement that surpasses all others. Without it, no amount of rules or techniques will have a significant impact. However, if you possess

this vital element, you can achieve remarkable results without relying solely on suggestions. So, what is this crucial requirement? It is a deep, unwavering desire to learn and a resolute determination to build your dream body.

How can you develop such an urge? By constantly reminding yourself of its immense importance. Envision the incredible transformation you seek, both in appearance and overall well-being. Embrace the vision of a vibrant, fulfilling, and joyful life.

Let this profound desire be your driving force, motivating you through challenges and setbacks. With this hunger for growth and transformation, you have the power to embark on an extraordinary journey of self-improvement. Embrace the power of your aspirations and let them guide you toward the body and life you've always dreamed of.

2. Approach this book with an open mind and curiosity. Be willing to challenge your current beliefs and explore new concepts. This book offers a wealth of knowledge and insights that may reshape your understanding of fitness and nutrition.

3. Keep a notebook or journal handy while reading. Take notes on key points, personal insights, and questions that arise in your mind. You can also underline a suggestion that you come across and think you can use.

4. Only knowledge that is used sticks in your mind. We learn by doing. As you progress through this book, start developing an action plan based on the strategies and recommendations provided. Break down your goals into actionable steps and apply the knowledge you get from this book as soon as possible. This will help you translate knowledge into practical application.

5. Apply the principles consistently, stay committed to your goals, and trust in the process. Remember that transforming your body and improving your health is a journey that requires patience. Results will come with time and dedication.

6. Regularly reflect on your progress, challenges, and successes. Adjust your approach if required and celebrate the milestones along the way. Think about what you have done wrong, what you can do better, and what you're satisfied with. Self-awareness and self-reflection are powerful tools for growth and continuous improvement.

7. Review this book each month. Go through your notes, the guidance you have underlined, and the key principles of this book. The human brain forgets things at an incredibly fast rate, so it's important to apply and remind yourself of the knowledge in this book.

8. Use this book as a catalyst for long-term lifestyle changes. The ultimate goal is to create lasting habits and build a self-image that supports your well-being and goals well beyond the pages of this book.

9. Before diving into the chapters, take some time to establish your goals. Whether it's building muscle, losing fat, improving performance, or enhancing overall health, having clear goals will help you apply the principles in this book more effectively.

To get the most out of this book:

a. Develop a deep, unwavering desire to build your dream body.

b. Approach this book with curiosity and an open mind.

c. Take notes and underline important ideas.

d. Apply the knowledge of this book at every opportunity and develop an action plan.

e. Practice patience and consistency.

f. Self-reflect and check up on the progress you are making each week. Ask yourself what improvements you have made, what mistakes, and what lessons you have learned for the future.

g. Review this book each month.

h. Embrace long-term lifestyle changes.

i. Establish your goals clearly.

II: Energy and Nutrition

Nutrition is the foundation of any successful fitness journey. Your diet plays a crucial role in supporting your body's physiological processes, providing energy for workouts, and aiding in muscle building and fat loss.

In the Energy and Nutrition chapter, we'll explore the fundamentals of a healthy and balanced diet, including the macronutrients (protein, carbohydrates, and fats) and micronutrients (vitamins and minerals) that your body needs to function optimally. We'll also discuss the importance of caloric balance and macronutrient ratios for achieving your fitness goals.

We'll then dive into the different types of diets and nutrition approaches that you can use to support your fitness goals, including high-protein diets, low-carb diets, and flexible dieting. We'll also touch on the benefits and potential drawbacks of different dietary approaches and how to choose the right approach for your needs.

Finally, we'll discuss practical tips for meal planning, food preparation, and eating on the go, as well as strategies for staying motivated and consistent with your nutrition plan. By the end of this chapter, you'll have a solid understanding of how to fuel your body for optimal health and fitness.

Energy and Fuel: Understanding Calories, Calorie Deficits, and Calorie Surpluses

When it comes to maintaining a healthy weight and fueling our bodies for optimal performance, understanding the role of calories is essential. A calorie is a unit of measurement that represents the amount of energy contained in food. Our bodies require a certain amount of calories each day to maintain basic bodily functions such as breathing and performing daily activities. This is known as our basal metabolic rate (BMR).

If you consume more calories than your body expends, you will gain weight. On the other hand, if you consume fewer calories than your body expends, you will lose weight. This is the basis of the concept of calorie deficits and calorie surpluses.

A calorie deficit occurs when we consume fewer calories than our body expends. It is often referred to as a "cut". This can be achieved through a combination of reducing calorie intake and increasing physical activity. When our body is in a calorie deficit, it must turn to stored energy (i.e. fat) to make up for the energy deficit. This results in weight loss. The size of the calorie deficit will determine the rate at which weight loss occurs. A deficit of 500 calories per day is generally recommended for a safe and sustainable rate of weight loss. To facilitate a calorie deficit sustainably, you need to first build good & healthy habits:

- Lean protein and veggies with every meal

- Less processed, nutrient-empty, and sugary foods

- Eating out less often (this allows you to directly control what you eat and the ingredients in your meal)

- Replacing calorie-dense liquids and foods with lower-calorie alternatives (e.g. instead of regular Coca-Cola, try the Zero version, or instead of a chocolate candy bar, try a protein bar).

- Consistent resistance training and cardio

- Quality sleep, recovery, and hydration.

A calorie surplus, on the other hand, occurs when we consume more calories than our body expends. This can result in weight gain. However, not all weight gain is necessarily bad - if the weight gain is due to an increase in muscle mass from strength training, for example, it can be beneficial. The key is to make sure that the calorie surplus is not too large and that the weight gain is primarily lean muscle mass. A recommended range for a calorie surplus is between 300-500 calories per day. This range allows for a healthy balance between gaining muscle mass and limiting the accumulation of body fat. It also ensures that the calorie surplus is not too low, which can impede muscle growth, while still promoting a sustainable rate of muscle gain.

Here are some habits, methods, and tips to help you reach your calorie surplus:

- Add fat to your meals. E.g., add olive oil to your salad or spaghetti sauce. I recommend adding oil to all your carbs. It doesn't take up much room in your stomach and is very calorie dense. Also, add fat to your protein shakes or smoothies. The best ones are peanut butter or whipping cream

- Eat your meals faster. You'll be able to eat more before your brain senses that you're full.

- Having high-calorie snacks like nuts or fruits will make it easier for you to hit your calorie goal. One handful of nuts (approximately 1 oz)

contains around 128-204 calories.

- Get used to feeling stuffed. Yes, you will get some discomfort from eating that much sometimes. But just as you have to get used to feeling hungry occasionally on a calorie deficit (cut), you will have to get used to eating when you don't want to while bulking.

It's important to note that not all calories are created equal. The types of foods we eat can have a significant impact on our health and weight management. For example, a calorie from a nutrient-dense whole food such as a piece of fruit will have a much different impact on our body than a calorie from a highly processed, sugar-laden snack due to the effects it has on our hormones and performance in the gym. In general, it's best to focus on consuming a diet rich in whole, nutrient-dense foods such as fruits, vegetables, whole grains, lean proteins, and healthy fats.

In addition to the quantity and quality of calories we consume, the timing of our meals can also play a role in weight management. Some people find success with intermittent fasting, which involves restricting food intake to a specific window of time each day. This can help to reduce overall calorie intake and promote weight loss. However, it's important to note that intermittent fasting is not appropriate for everyone and should be done under the guidance of a healthcare professional.

In conclusion, understanding the role of calories in our body is essential for maintaining a healthy weight and fueling our bodies for optimal performance. By consuming the right quantity and quality of calories, and timing our meals appropriately, we can achieve our weight management goals and improve our overall health and well-being.

Energy from food is measured in calories or joules. One calorie equals 4.184 joules

Energy in terms of food and nutrition is defined as the energy released from carbohydrates, proteins, fats, and fibers. It is measured in calories/kilocalories (kcal) or joules/kilojoules (kJ).

Macronutrients & Micronutrients

Protein, fat, fiber, and carbohydrates (often called carbs) are all macronutrients. Macronutrients are the nutrients we need in large quantities that provide us with energy. 1 gram of protein contains 4 calories, 1 gram of fat provides 9 calories and 1 gram of carbs contains 4 calories.

Micronutrients are the essential vitamins and minerals required by our bodies in small quantities to maintain good health. While macronutrients like carbohydrates, proteins, and fats get more attention in the diet, micronutrients are just as crucial to overall health and wellness.

There are several different types of micronutrients that the body needs, including vitamins A, B, C, D, E, and K, as well as minerals like iron, calcium, magnesium, and zinc. Each of these micronutrients plays a unique role in maintaining optimal health.

For example, vitamin C is essential for maintaining a healthy immune system and preventing infections and diseases, while vitamin D helps the body absorb calcium and maintain strong bones and teeth. Iron is important for oxygen transport and preventing anemia, and calcium is vital for bone health and preventing osteoporosis.

While most people can get all the necessary micronutrients through a balanced diet, some individuals may need to supplement their intake with vitamins and minerals. This could be due to dietary restrictions, health conditions, or lifestyle factors.

It's important to note that getting too much of certain micronutrients can also be harmful to the body. For example, excessive intake of vitamin A can lead to toxicity, while high levels of iron can cause damage to the liver and other organs.

To ensure that you're getting the right amount of micronutrients, it's important to speak with a healthcare professional or registered dietitian. They can help assess your individual needs and recommend any necessary supplements or dietary changes.

While micronutrients may be small, they are mighty in their importance for overall health and wellness. It's important to prioritize a balanced diet that includes a variety of nutrient-rich foods to ensure you're getting all the necessary vitamins and minerals your body needs. Micronutrients do not contain any significant calories. While macronutrients such as carbohydrates, fats, and proteins are the primary sources of calories in our diets, micronutrients like vitamins and minerals do not contribute significantly to calorie intake. These essential nutrients are required by the body in small amounts for various functions such as metabolism, growth, repair of tissues, and maintaining overall health and well-being. Consuming excessive amounts of micronutrients beyond the recommended daily intake can lead to adverse health effects rather than providing any nutritional benefits.

Protein

Our body's muscle tissue is built up of protein. We need protein for our muscles to function, recover and grow. If you do not consume enough protein, your muscle will start to break down, you will lose strength and muscle size. Protein is an essential nutrient for building and repairing muscle tissue. When you exercise, especially with resistance training, you create small tears in your muscle fibers. Protein is required to repair and rebuild these fibers, which ultimately leads to muscle growth.

In addition to its role in muscle repair and growth, protein also plays a crucial role in regulating various physiological processes in the body, such as hormone production, immune function, and nutrient transport.

For optimal muscle growth, it's recommended to consume between 1.8-2.2 grams of protein per kilogram of body weight per day. This can be challenging to achieve through whole food sources alone, which is why many people turn to protein supplements like whey protein powder.

The rate at which our bodies can absorb and utilize protein is a topic of ongoing research and debate. While individual factors and specific circumstances can influence protein absorption, current scientific evidence suggests that our bodies can effectively absorb and utilize approximately 20-30 grams of protein per meal.

Protein absorption is a complex process that involves digestion, breakdown into amino acids, and uptake into the bloodstream. The rate of absorption can vary depending on several factors, including the source and type of protein, the presence of other nutrients, and individual factors such as age, metabolic rate, and overall health.

Consuming a moderate amount of protein per meal, within the range of 20-30 grams, appears to maximize muscle protein synthesis—the process responsible for muscle repair and growth. This range allows for optimal stimulation of muscle protein synthesis without significantly exceeding the body's capacity to absorb and utilize the amino acids.

It's important to note that protein absorption is not an all-or-nothing process. Consuming large amounts of protein in a single meal doesn't necessarily mean that the excess protein will go to waste. The body can store and utilize amino acids over time. However, spreading protein intake evenly throughout the day, across multiple meals and snacks, may provide a more consistent and sustained supply of amino acids for muscle protein synthesis.

Individual protein needs can vary based on factors such as body weight, activity level, and specific goals.

Consuming excessive amounts of protein won't necessarily lead to more muscle growth, as the body can only utilize so much protein at once. Consuming too much protein can also place unnecessary stress on the kidneys and potentially lead to health complications.

Protein is a crucial nutrient for building and repairing muscle tissue, as well as regulating various physiological processes in the body. Aim to consume an adequate amount of protein each day through a combination of whole food sources and supplements, while avoiding excessive intake.

Protein is made up of amino acids. Roughly 500 different amino acids have been identified in nature, but just 20 amino acids make up the proteins in the human body. These 20 amino acids are classified into two groups; essential amino acids (EAAs) and non-essential amino acids.

Out of the 20 amino acids, 9 of them are essential amino acids, and the rest of them are non-essential amino acids.

Essential amino acids (EAAS), also known as indispensable amino acids are amino acids that we humans cannot synthesize in our bodies, which means they must be supplied through our diet. The best sources of amino acids are found in animal proteins such as meat, eggs, milk, etc. These proteins are complete, meaning they contain all of the 9 essential amino acids our body needs. Some plant-based foods also contain all the 9 essential amino acids, e.g. buckwheat, hemp seeds, chia seeds, and spirulina. Before explaining the major problem with plant protein let's first list all the 20 amino acids that make up the proteins in the human body.

Essential amino acids

Branched-chain amino acids

Branched-chain amino acids (aka. BCAA) are a group of 3 essential amino acids: valine, leucine, and isoleucine. These amino acids have a molecular structure with a branch. BCAAs are important for muscle growth and repair due to their plentifulness in muscle protein. BCAAs also provide energy during exercise. BCAAs are most commonly found in complete protein-rich foods such as meat, dairy, chicken, fish, and eggs. For vegans, nutritional sources of BCAAs in smaller amounts include lentils, nuts, and soy proteins.

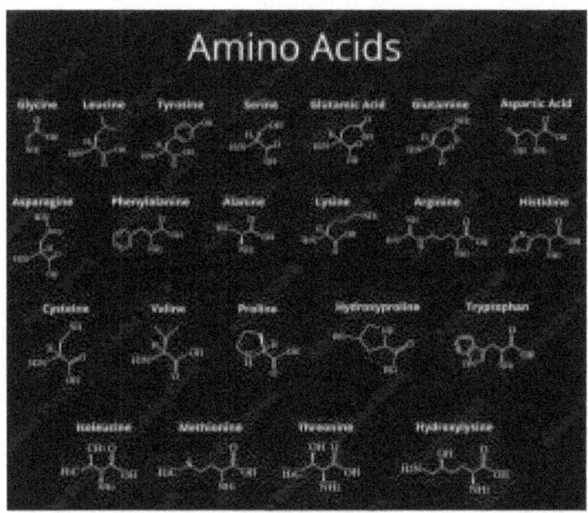

Lysine

Lysine is an essential amino acid that is frequently mentioned due to its crucial role in protein synthesis and other bodily functions. Although lysine is found in a variety of foods, staples such as bread and rice are low in this nutrient. For instance, wheat, which is a common source of protein for people in developing countries, has a suboptimal amino acid profile and is particularly low in lysine.

Consequently, a lack of lysine and other essential amino acids in the diet can result in serious health complications, such as stunted growth for teenagers and impaired immune function. This issue is especially prevalent in developing countries where people may rely heavily on a single source of protein, such as wheat, to meet their nutritional needs. As previously said, animal proteins are complete proteins and contain all of the 9 essential amino acids our body needs, thus it also contains lysine. Foods that naturally contain the most lysine are:

- Meat, specifically red meat, and pork.

- Cheese, particularly Parmesan

- Fish, e.g. cod and sardines

- Eggs

Some of the Vegan options that contain lysine (in fewer amounts than animal proteins) are:

- Soybeans, particularly tofu or isolated soy protein.

- Spirulina

- Fenugreek seed

Threonine

Threonine plays an important role in numerous biological processes, including protein synthesis, immune function, and the maintenance of healthy skin, bones, and teeth. It is also involved in the synthesis of neurotransmitters, which are chemicals that transmit signals in the nervous system.

Threonine is found in a wide range of foods, including meat, fish, poultry, eggs, beans, nuts, and seeds. However, the threonine content of plant-based foods tends to be lower than that of animal-based foods. As a result, vegetarians and vegans may need to pay close attention to their threonine intake to ensure that they are meeting their daily requirements.

A deficiency of threonine can result in a range of health problems, including weakness, fatigue, and irritability. In severe cases, threonine deficiency can lead to impaired immune function, digestive disorders, and other serious health complications.

On the other hand, excessive consumption of threonine is rare, as excess amounts are usually excreted by the body. However, very high doses of threonine supplements may cause stomach upset, nausea, and other adverse effects. As with any dietary supplement, it is important to consult a healthcare professional before taking threonine or any other amino acid supplement.

Phenylalanine

This amino acid plays a crucial role in the production of other amino acids, neurotransmitters such as dopamine and norepinephrine, and important proteins.

There are three forms of phenylalanine: L-phenylalanine, D-phenylalanine, and DL-phenylalanine. L-phenylalanine is the most common form found in foods and is used by the body to make proteins. D-phenylalanine, on the other hand, is not used by the body to make proteins and is often used as an alternative therapy for chronic pain or depression. DL-phenylalanine is a combination of L-phenylalanine and D-phenylalanine and is used for similar purposes as D-phenylalanine.

While phenylalanine is generally safe for most people, high doses can be harmful, especially in individuals with phenylketonuria (PKU), a genetic disorder that prevents the body from breaking down phenylalanine properly. PKU is usually diagnosed in infancy and requires strict dietary restrictions to prevent brain damage and other complications.

Phenylalanine is found in a variety of foods, including:

1. Meat and poultry (such as beef, chicken, and turkey).

2. Fish (such as salmon, tuna, and halibut).

3. Dairy products (such as milk, cheese, and yogurt).

4. Soy products (such as tofu, soy milk, and soybeans).

5. Nuts and seeds (such as almonds, peanuts, and pumpkin seeds).

6. Legumes (such as lentils and chickpeas).

7. Vegetables (such as spinach, kale, and broccoli).

Phenylalanine is also available in supplement form and is frequently combined with other amino acids, vitamins, or minerals to promote its absorption and efficacy. However, it is important to talk to a healthcare provider before taking any supplements to determine the appropriate dosage and ensure they are safe for your specific needs.

Methionine

Methionine is important for several critical functions in the body, such as the development of healthy skin, nails, and hair, the formation of cartilage tissue, and the metabolism of fats.

Methionine is found in a variety of foods, including:

1. Meat, poultry, and fish (such as beef, chicken, salmon, and tuna).

2. Dairy products (such as milk, cheese, and yogurt).

3. Eggs.

4. Nuts and seeds (such as Brazil nuts, sesame seeds, and sunflower seeds).

5. Legumes (such as lentils, chickpeas, and kidney beans).

6. Whole grains (such as oats, rice, and quinoa).

While methionine is generally safe for most people, high doses can be harmful, especially in individuals with certain medical conditions, such as kidney disease. In addition, some studies suggest that high levels of methionine in the diet may increase the risk of certain health problems, such as heart disease and cancer. However, more research is needed in this area to fully understand the relationship between methionine intake and disease risk.

Histidine

This amino acid plays a vital role in the growth and repair of tissues in the body as well as in the production of red and white blood cells. Additionally, histidine acts as a precursor for histamine, a neurotransmitter that helps regulate immune responses, digestion, and sleep-wake cycles.

Histidine is found in many foods, including:

1. Poultry (such as chicken and turkey).

2. Fish (such as tuna, salmon, and halibut).

3. Meat (such as beef and pork).

4. Dairy products (such as milk, cheese, and yogurt).

5. Eggs.

6. Nuts and seeds (such as pumpkin and sesame seeds).

Symptoms of histidine deficiency are rare, but they can include anemia, delayed growth and development in children, and changes in mood or cognitive function. Histidine supplements may be recommended for people with certain disorders, like rheumatoid arthritis, but always consult a healthcare provider before taking supplements to ensure they are safe and appropriate for your needs.

Tryptophan

Tryptophan is a precursor to the neurotransmitter serotonin, which regulates mood, appetite, and sleep. Additionally, tryptophan is used by the body to produce niacin, an essential B vitamin.

Tryptophan is found in many foods, including:

1. Poultry (such as chicken and turkey).

2. Fish (such as salmon and halibut).

3. Dairy products (such as milk, cheese, and yogurt).

4. Eggs.

5. Nuts and seeds (such as pumpkin and sesame seeds).

6. Legumes (such as soybeans, lentils, and chickpeas).

7. Grains (such as oats, quinoa, and rice).

While tryptophan is generally safe for most people, it can sometimes interact with other medications or supplements, so it is essential to talk to a healthcare provider before taking any supplements. It is also important to note that tryptophan supplements can cause some side effects, such as gastrointestinal issues or drowsiness.

Non-essential amino acids

Glutamine

Glutamine is an amino acid, which is one of the building blocks of proteins. It is a nonessential amino acid, which means that the body can produce it on its own, but it can also be obtained from dietary sources. Glutamine is found in a wide variety of foods, including meat, fish, dairy products, beans, and vegetables.

Glutamine plays several important roles in the body. It is involved in the synthesis of proteins, the regulation of acid-base balance, and the transport of nitrogen between tissues. Glutamine is also an important source of energy for many types of cells, including immune cells and cells in the lining of the intestine.

To clarify, glutamine supplementation may be beneficial in certain situations, such as for people with gastrointestinal disorders or athletes and individuals undergoing intense physical training. However, for the average person who is consuming a balanced diet, supplementation may not be necessary. It is important to consult with a healthcare professional before beginning any supplementation regimen. While glutamine can help reduce muscle soreness and improve exercise performance in some cases, it is important to note that excessive intake can be harmful, particularly for people with liver or kidney disease. Additionally, a diet that is already rich in protein may provide sufficient amounts of glutamine, making supplementation unnecessary and a waste of money.

Aspartate

Aspartate, also known as aspartic acid, is an amino acid that is found in both plants and animals.

Aspartate is found in many different types of foods, including meat, fish, dairy products, and certain vegetables such as asparagus and beets. It is also commonly used as a food additive, particularly in the form of monosodium glutamate (MSG).

In the body, aspartate plays many important roles. It is involved in the synthesis of proteins, as well as in the production of other amino acids such as asparagine and arginine. Aspartate is also a key component of the citric acid cycle, which is a series of biochemical reactions that produce energy in cells.

In addition to its role in metabolism, aspartate has been studied for its potential health benefits. Some research suggests that it may help to reduce fatigue and improve athletic performance. It has also been investigated for its potential role in treating certain neurological disorders, including Alzheimer's disease and epilepsy. However, more research is needed to fully understand the effects of aspartate on these conditions. A reminder that before you take anything you should consult a healthcare professional.

Glutamate

Glutamate is an amino acid that acts as an excitatory neurotransmitter in the central nervous system (CNS). It is the most abundant neurotransmitter in the brain and is involved in many important physiological processes, including learning, memory, and synaptic plasticity.

Glutamate is found in many foods, particularly in protein-rich foods such as meats, fish, and dairy products. It is also commonly used as a flavor enhancer and food additive, and is found in many processed foods under the name "monosodium glutamate" or "MSG".

In the brain, glutamate is synthesized by neurons and released into the synapse, where it binds to glutamate receptors on the postsynaptic membrane. There are several types of glutamate receptors, including NMDA receptors, AMPA receptors, and kainate receptors, which play important roles in synaptic transmission and plasticity.

Excessive glutamate release or impaired glutamate uptake can lead to excitotoxicity, a process in which excessive levels of glutamate cause damage to neurons and contribute to various neurological disorders such as stroke, traumatic brain injury, and neurodegenerative diseases like Alzheimer's and Parkinson's disease.

On the other hand, drugs that enhance glutamate signaling, such as NMDA receptor agonists, have been shown to have cognitive-enhancing effects and are being explored as potential treatments for cognitive dysfunction and neurodegenerative diseases.

Arginine

Arginine is an amino acid that is often used in fitness supplements due to its ability to increase blood flow and promote the production of nitric oxide in the body. Nitric oxide is a molecule that helps to dilate blood vessels and improve circulation, which can potentially enhance athletic performance and improve muscle recovery.

In particular, arginine is often used by athletes and bodybuilders to improve their muscle pumps during workouts. A muscle pump is the feeling of tightness and fullness that occurs in the muscles during exercise and is thought to be related to increased blood flow and nutrient delivery to the muscles. By promoting blood flow and nitric oxide production, arginine may be able to enhance the muscle pump and promote muscle growth.

Arginine has also been shown to have potential benefits for endurance athletes, as it may improve the delivery of oxygen and nutrients to the muscles during prolonged exercise. Additionally, arginine has been shown to have antioxidant properties, which may help to protect the body from the oxidative stress that can occur during intense exercise.

Overall, while the evidence for the benefits of arginine in fitness is somewhat mixed, it is a popular ingredient in many pre-workout and muscle-building supplements due to its potential effects on blood flow and muscle pumps.

Arginine is an amino acid that is naturally found in a wide variety of foods, including both plant and animal sources. Some of the best dietary sources of arginine include:

- Meat: Beef, pork, chicken, and turkey are all good sources of arginine.

- Fish: Many types of fish, including salmon, tuna, and halibut, contain high levels of arginine.

- Dairy: Milk, cheese, and yogurt are all good sources of arginine.

- Nuts and seeds: Almonds, peanuts, walnuts, and sesame seeds are all rich in arginine.

- Legumes: Soybeans, lentils, and chickpeas are all good sources of arginine.

- Whole grains: Whole wheat, oats, and quinoa all contain significant amounts of arginine.

Arginine is also available in supplement form, both as a standalone product and as an ingredient in pre-workout and muscle-building supplements. However, it is generally recommended to obtain nutrients from whole foods rather than relying on supplements whenever possible.

Alanine

Alanine is a non-essential amino acid, meaning that it can be synthesized by the body and does not need to be obtained through the diet. It is involved in a variety of metabolic processes in the body and has been studied for its potential role in fitness and athletic performance.

One of the primary benefits of alanine in fitness is its role in buffering lactic acid buildup in the muscles. During intense exercise, the body produces lactic acid as a byproduct of anaerobic metabolism. This buildup of lactic acid can cause fatigue and a burning sensation in the muscles, which can limit athletic performance. Alanine can help to buffer this buildup of lactic acid, which may enhance endurance and delay the onset of fatigue during exercise.

Alanine is also involved in the production of glucose in the liver, which can be important for maintaining blood sugar levels during exercise. During prolonged exercise, the body may begin to break down muscle tissue as a source of energy, which can lead to muscle loss and decreased athletic performance. However, by supporting the production of glucose in the liver, alanine may help to prevent this muscle breakdown and maintain energy levels during exercise.

Alanine is found in a variety of protein-rich foods, including meat, poultry, fish, dairy products, and eggs. It can also be synthesized by the body from other amino acids, such as glutamate. While alanine supplements are available, they are generally not necessary for most people, as the body can synthesize sufficient amounts of alanine on its own.

Proline

Proline is an amino acid that is important in the formation of collagen, which is a key component of connective tissue such as tendons, ligaments, and cartilage. It is also involved in the maintenance of healthy skin, joints, and muscles.

In terms of fitness, proline can be beneficial for athletes and fitness enthusiasts because it helps to maintain healthy joints and connective tissue, which is especially important for activities that put stress on the joints, such as weightlifting, running, and other high-impact activities.

Proline can be found in a variety of dietary sources, including meat, dairy products, eggs, and some plant-based sources such as soybeans, wheat germ, and mushrooms. It can also be synthesized by the body from other amino acids, although the rate of synthesis is relatively low.

Cysteine

Cysteine is a sulfur-containing amino acid that plays several important roles in the body. It is a key component of the antioxidant glutathione and is also involved in the synthesis of proteins, the maintenance of healthy skin and hair, and the maintenance of the immune system.

In terms of fitness, cysteine may be beneficial due to its role in antioxidant defense. Exercise can generate free radicals, which can cause oxidative damage to cells and tissues. Antioxidants such as cysteine help to neutralize these free radicals and protect against oxidative stress.

Cysteine can be found in a variety of dietary sources, including meat, poultry, fish, eggs, dairy products, nuts, and seeds. It can also be synthesized by the body from other amino acids, although the rate of synthesis is relatively low. Additionally, cysteine is available as a dietary supplement in various forms, including N-acetylcysteine (NAC), which is commonly used to support immune function and respiratory health. However, it is important to note that excessive intake of cysteine or its supplements may be harmful, and should be avoided without medical guidance.

Asparagine

Asparagine is a non-essential amino acid, meaning that it can be synthesized by the human body. It is important for the proper functioning of the nervous system and the immune system and is also involved in the synthesis of proteins.

Although it was initially discovered in asparagus, asparagine is found in a variety of dietary sources, including meat, fish, eggs, dairy products, nuts, seeds, and certain vegetables such as asparagus, potatoes, and legumes.

Asparagine is closely associated with the tricarboxylic acid (TCA) cycle, which is a series of chemical reactions that occur in the mitochondria of cells and are involved in the production of energy. Asparagine is converted to aspartate, an important intermediary in the TCA cycle. This means that asparagine is indirectly involved in energy production in the body.

It is important to note that while asparagine is not considered an essential amino acid, meaning that it does not need to be obtained through the diet, it may become conditionally essential in certain circumstances, such as during periods of rapid growth or recovery from injury or illness. In these cases, supplementation with asparagine or its precursors may be beneficial.

Serine

Serine is an amino acid that is found in many proteins and is involved in various metabolic processes in the body. In terms of fitness, serine plays a role in muscle growth and repair, as well as in the production of energy during exercise.

Serine is found in many different foods, including meat, poultry, fish, dairy products, nuts, seeds, and legumes. It can also be synthesized in the body from other amino acids, such as glycine.

One of the key roles of serine in fitness is its involvement in the biosynthesis of creatine, which is an important compound for muscle growth and energy production. Creatine is synthesized in the liver and kidneys from arginine, glycine, and methionine, with serine playing a critical role in the conversion of glycine to creatine.

Serine is also involved in the production of ATP, which is the primary source of energy for muscle contractions during exercise. It is a precursor to phosphatidylserine, which is a component of cell membranes and is involved in the transport of nutrients and waste products in and out of cells.

In summary, serine is an important amino acid for fitness because it plays a role in muscle growth and repair, as well as in the production of energy during exercise. It is found in many different foods, and can also be synthesized in the body from other amino acids.

Glycine

Glycine is the simplest amino acid, with only a hydrogen atom as its side chain. Glycine is found in high concentrations in collagen, which is a major component of connective tissue, and also plays important roles in various metabolic processes in the body.

In terms of fitness, glycine is involved in synthesizing creatine, compound for muscle growth and energy production. Glycine is one of the three amino acids required for the biosynthesis of creatine, along with arginine and methionine. Creatine is synthesized in the liver and kidneys and is used by muscle cells to produce energy during intense exercise.

Glycine is also important for the synthesis of glutathione, which is a powerful antioxidant that helps protect cells from oxidative stress. Glutathione is synthesized from three amino acids, including glycine, and plays a critical role in detoxifying harmful substances in the body.

Additionally, glycine is involved in the production of collagen, which is a key component of tendons, ligaments, and cartilage. Collagen provides structural support to these tissues and helps maintain their strength and flexibility.

Glycine is found in high concentrations in protein-rich foods such as meat, poultry, fish, dairy products, and legumes. It can also be synthesized in the body from other amino acids, such as serine and threonine.

In summary, glycine is an important amino acid for fitness because it is involved in the synthesis of creatine, which is important for muscle growth and energy production, as well as the synthesis of glutathione, which helps protect cells from oxidative stress. It is also important for the production of collagen, which provides structural support to tendons, ligaments, and cartilage.

Tyrosine

Tyrosine is an amino acid that plays an important role in the body's production of neurotransmitters, including dopamine, epinephrine, and norepinephrine. These neurotransmitters are involved in regulating mood, motivation, and energy levels, among other functions.

In the context of fitness, some people use tyrosine supplements in an attempt to improve exercise performance, increase focus and motivation during workouts, and reduce fatigue. However, the evidence supporting these effects is mixed and more research is needed to determine the effectiveness of tyrosine supplements for improving exercise performance.

Tyrosine is found naturally in a variety of foods, including meat, fish, dairy products, nuts, and seeds. It can also be synthesized in the body from another amino acid called phenylalanine. Therefore, most people can obtain sufficient amounts of tyrosine through their diet and do not need to supplement with it. As with any supplement, it is important to talk to a healthcare provider before taking tyrosine supplements, especially if you have any medical conditions or are taking medications.

Why Protein Quality Matters (The Issue With Plant Protein)

Let's talk about the differences between plant protein and animal protein and why the quality of protein matters. Our body absorbs and utilizes certain proteins better than others, and the quality of a protein source is measured by a score called DIAAS (Digestible Indispensable Amino Acid Score). Animal proteins such as cow's milk, eggs, beef, and chicken breast are considered high-quality proteins because they are easily digestible and contain all the essential amino acids that our body needs.

On the other hand, plant protein sources such as vegan protein powders, chickpeas, quinoa, and buckwheat, are considered "good quality" proteins but fall lower on the DIAAS score than animal proteins. Some plant proteins, such as rice, lentils, nuts, and wheat, are considered poor-quality sources of protein. Although you can still hit your daily protein goals with plant-based sources, research shows that protein quality matters, and some plant proteins may not provide enough of one or more essential amino acids.

Protein quality is essential for our body's growth and development. A study of men's height in 105 countries found that protein quality, as well as quantity, played a crucial role in their height. Another study found that children and teenagers who didn't eat meat were shorter and had weaker bones. This shows that protein quality comes down to amino acids, and our body needs all the essential amino acids to build and maintain muscle mass.

It's important to note that the protein you eat isn't necessarily the same as the protein your body utilizes. Eating 40 grams of protein from lentils may result in your body utilizing only around 21 grams of protein due to their DIAAS score of 54%. In contrast, consuming the same amount of protein from animal sources with a DIAAS score of 100% or more would result in your body utilizing more protein.

It's crucial to meet your daily protein requirements, and for people who don't resistance train or are trying to build muscle, the recommended minimum protein intake is at least 1.2-1.6g (around 2g for people who want to build muscle) per kg of body weight. With the right knowledge and diligence, it's possible to meet protein requirements with a vegan or vegetarian diet, but it's essential to choose the right protein sources to ensure adequate utilization and absorption.

Food Item	Food Group	DIAAS Value (%)
Dry milk	Dairy	144
Bacon (smoked-cooked)	Pork	142
Milk protein concentrate	Dairy	141
Pork loin (medium)	Pork	139
Whey protein concentrate	Dairy	133
Ham (alternatively-cured)	Pork	133
Ribeye (roast, medium)	Beef	130
Bologna	Pork	128
Ham (conventionally-cured)	Pork	126
Whey protein isolate	Dairy	125
Ham (non-cured)	Pork	124
Skimmed milk powder	Dairy	123
Eggs	Eggs	122
Ground beef (raw)	Beef	121
Beef jerky	Beef	120
Salami	Pork	120
Pork belly (raw)	Pork	119
Milk protein concentrate	Dairy	118
Pork loin (medium-well done)	Pork	118
Bacon (smoked)	Pork	117
Pork loin (well-done)	Pork	117
Ribeye (roast, medium-rare)	Beef	111
Whey protein isolate	Dairy	109
Ribeye (well-done)	Beef	107
Soy flour	Legumes	105

In protein form (food or powder) it takes three to four hours for our body to absorb amino acids. When consumed in a crystalline (powder) form, amino acids can be absorbed by the body in as little as 30 minutes. This makes them an ideal source of nutrition for sports and training as they can be consumed precisely when the body requires them.

As long as your daily protein intake is sufficient and your diet includes a diverse range of proteins that includes animal-based sources, I advise against taking any additional amino acid supplements e.g. EAAs or BCAAs. Consuming an adequate amount of protein from whole food sources such as meat and eggs provides the essential amino acids that are necessary for your body's needs and optimal muscle function and growth.

Amino acid supplementations can be particularly beneficial for individuals following a vegan diet. As vegan diets exclude all animal-based food sources, certain essential amino acids, vitamins, and minerals that are vital for our bodies and muscles may be missed. To compensate for these deficiencies, the best option for vegans is to use a vegan protein powder or EAA powder to supplement these important micronutrients and amino acids.

The Importance Of Protein For Building Muscle And Losing Fat

Protein plays a crucial role in muscle building and is often referred to as the "building block" of muscles. Understanding the importance of protein for muscle growth is essential for anyone looking to achieve their fitness goals. Here's why protein is vital for muscle building:

1. Muscle Repair and Growth: During exercise, especially resistance training, small tears occur in your muscle fibers. Protein provides the necessary amino acids to repair and rebuild these damaged muscle tissues. It supports muscle recovery and promotes the growth of new muscle fibers, leading to increased muscle size and strength.

2. Protein Synthesis: Muscle protein synthesis is the process by which the body assembles new proteins within the muscle fibers. Adequate protein intake stimulates muscle protein synthesis, ensuring that the rate of muscle protein synthesis exceeds or matches the rate of breakdown. This creates a positive muscle protein balance, leading to muscle growth over time.

3. Muscle Preservation: Protein intake is crucial for preserving existing muscle mass. When you're in a calorie deficit or engaging in intense physical activity, your body may break down muscle protein for energy. Sufficient protein consumption helps minimize muscle breakdown, preserving your hard-earned muscle and preventing muscle loss.

4. Strength and Performance: Protein not only contributes to muscle growth but also enhances strength and athletic performance. As your muscles grow stronger and more resilient through protein synthesis, you'll experience improved power, endurance, and overall physical

performance. This is particularly important for athletes and individuals engaged in strength or endurance training.

5. Thermic Effect and Satiety: Protein has a higher thermic effect compared to carbohydrates and fats, meaning it requires more energy for digestion and absorption. This increases your metabolism and can contribute to additional calorie expenditure. Additionally, protein-rich meals promote feelings of fullness and satiety, helping you control your appetite and manage calorie intake.

6. Nutrient Density: Protein-rich foods often come with additional essential nutrients, such as vitamins, minerals, and antioxidants. These nutrients support overall health, aid in muscle recovery, and promote optimal bodily functions. Including a variety of high-quality protein sources, such as lean meats, fish, eggs, dairy, legumes, and plant-based options, ensures a well-rounded and nutrient-dense diet.

7. Individual Protein Needs: It's important to consider individual protein requirements based on factors like age, gender, body composition, activity level, and goals. While recommended protein intake may vary, a general guideline for active individuals is to aim for approximately 0.8-1 gram of protein per pound of body weight (or 1.8-2.2 grams per kilogram).

In conclusion, protein is essential for muscle building as it supports muscle repair, stimulates protein synthesis, preserves muscle mass, enhances strength and performance, aids in weight management, and provides important nutrients for overall health. Incorporating protein-rich foods into your diet is key to unlocking your muscle-building potential and achieving your desired physique. Remember to combine protein intake with appropriate exercise and recovery strategies for optimal results.

Carbohydrates

Carbohydrates are one of the three macronutrients, alongside protein and fat, that are essential for our body's functions. Carbs are the body's primary source of energy, providing fuel for daily activities and exercise. There are different types of carbs, and not all of them are created equal. In this chapter, we'll take a closer look at what carbohydrates are, the different types of carbohydrates, and how they affect our health.

What are Carbohydrates?

Carbohydrates are one of the primary macronutrients that our bodies use for energy. They are molecules made up of carbon, hydrogen, and oxygen atoms. Carbs come in various forms, including simple and complex carbs, which are defined by their chemical structure and how quickly they are broken down and absorbed by the body.

Types of Carbohydrates:

1. Simple Carbohydrates:

Simple carbs are made up of one or two sugar molecules and are quickly absorbed into the bloodstream. Examples include table sugar, fruit, and honey. These types of carbs provide a quick burst of energy, but the energy is usually short-lived, leading to a "sugar crash" soon after consumption.

2. Complex Carbohydrates:

Complex carbs, on the other hand, are made up of three or more sugar molecules and take longer to break down and digest. Examples include whole grains, beans, and vegetables. These types of carbs provide a more sustained release of energy and can keep you feeling full for longer.

3. Fiber:

Fiber is a type of carbohydrate that cannot be digested by the body. It is found in plant-based foods such as fruits, vegetables, and whole grains. Fiber helps regulate digestion, keeps us feeling full, and can lower the risk of chronic diseases such as heart disease and diabetes.

How Carbohydrates Affect Our Health:

1. Energy:

As mentioned earlier, carbohydrates are the primary source of energy for our bodies. When we eat carbs, our bodies break them down into glucose, which is then used for energy. Without enough carbs in our diet, our bodies may turn to break down muscle tissue for energy, leading to muscle loss and fatigue.

2. Blood Sugar:

Eating too many simple carbs can cause spikes in blood sugar levels, which can be detrimental to our health. When we eat simple carbs, our bodies rapidly absorb them into the bloodstream, causing a quick rise in blood sugar levels. This can lead to insulin resistance, a precursor to type 2 diabetes.

3. Weight Management:

Carbs can play a significant role in weight management. While it's not necessary to cut out all carbs to lose weight, it's important to choose the right types of carbs. Complex carbs and fiber can keep us feeling full for longer, reducing our overall calorie intake. On the other hand, consuming too many simple carbs can lead to overeating and weight gain. When it comes to carbohydrate consumption, it's important to focus on quality rather than quantity. While all carbohydrates can provide energy, some sources are more nutrient-dense than others. For example, whole grains, fruits, and vegetables provide not only carbohydrates but also essential vitamins, minerals, and fiber, while added sugars and refined grains provide empty calories with little nutritional value.

Carbohydrates are an essential macronutrient that our bodies need for energy and proper function. However, not all carbs are created equal. Simple carbs can provide a quick burst of energy but are usually short-lived, while complex carbs and fiber can provide a sustained release of energy and keep us feeling full for longer. When it comes to carbohydrates, moderation is key. Choosing the right types of carbs and monitoring our intake can help us maintain good health. Also, carbohydrates are not obligatory. You can gain muscle and lose fat just as well without them as with them.

Fat

Fat is another essential macronutrient that the body needs to function properly. Like carbohydrates, fats are a source of energy, providing 9 calories per gram. However, unlike carbohydrates, the body can store fat for long periods, making it an important source of energy during prolonged periods of low food intake.

Dietary fats are broken down into smaller components called fatty acids, which are then absorbed into the bloodstream and utilized by the body. Additionally, the body can also produce fatty acids by converting carbohydrates from food. These fatty acids are essential for the production of various types of fats that the body requires to function properly.

In addition to being an energy source, fats also play a critical role in the body's hormonal and cellular functions. Fats are essential for the production of hormones, including sex hormones, and help to maintain healthy skin, hair, and nails.

There are three main types of dietary fats: saturated, unsaturated, and trans fats. Saturated fats are typically solid at room temperature and are found in animal products like meat and dairy as well as some plant-based sources like coconut oil. These fats have been linked to an increased risk of heart disease and should be consumed in moderation.

Unsaturated fats, on the other hand, are typically liquid at room temperature and can be found in foods like nuts, seeds, avocados, and fatty fish. These fats are important for heart health and can help lower cholesterol levels.

Trans fats are a type of fat created through a process called hydrogenation, which turns liquid oils into solid fats. These fats have been linked to an increased risk of heart disease and should be avoided as much as possible.

It's important to note that not all fats are created equal. When it comes to including fats in your diet, it's important to focus on healthy sources of fat, like those found in nuts, seeds, and fatty fish. Incorporating healthy fats into your diet can help improve overall health and prevent chronic diseases like heart disease and type 2 diabetes.

Like with carbohydrates, it's important to pay attention to the amount of fat you consume. While fat is an essential nutrient, consuming too much of it can lead to fat gain and increase your risk of chronic diseases. Aim to consume healthy sources of fat in moderation as part of a balanced diet.

The Role and Importance of Fats & Carbohydrates in Your Diet

Carbohydrates and fats are two essential macronutrients that play crucial roles in your diet and overall health. Understanding their functions and incorporating them appropriately into your eating plan is essential for a balanced and sustainable approach to nutrition. Let's explore the roles of carbohydrates and fats in your diet:

Carbohydrates:

Carbohydrates are your body's primary source of energy. They are broken down into glucose, which is used by your cells for fuel. Here's why carbohydrates are important:

1. Energy Source: Carbohydrates provide the energy your body needs to perform daily activities, exercise, and support bodily functions. Glucose is readily available and easily converted into

energy, making carbohydrates vital for fueling your muscles and brain.

2. Brain Function: Glucose derived from carbohydrates is the preferred fuel for your brain. Adequate carbohydrate intake ensures optimal brain function, including cognitive processes, concentration, and memory.

3. Exercise Performance: Carbohydrates are essential for high-intensity exercise and endurance activities. They provide quick energy to power your muscles during workouts and help sustain performance over extended periods. Glycogen, the stored form of glucose in your muscles and liver, is vital for athletic performance.

4. Nutrient Density: Carbohydrate-rich foods, such as fruits, vegetables, whole grains, and legumes, provide essential vitamins, minerals, fiber, and antioxidants. These nutrients support overall health, digestion, and disease prevention.

When incorporating carbohydrates into your diet, focus on whole, unprocessed sources. Opt for complex carbohydrates like whole grains, vegetables, fruits, and legumes, which provide sustained energy and essential nutrients. Limit refined carbohydrates like sugary snacks, pastries, and processed grains, as they offer fewer nutrients and can cause rapid blood sugar spikes.

Fats:

Fats are another essential macronutrient that serves several important functions in your body. Here's why fats are important in your diet:

1. Energy and Satiety: Fats are a concentrated source of energy, providing more than twice the calories per gram compared to carbohydrates and proteins. Including healthy fats in your diet helps

provide sustained energy and promotes feelings of fullness and satisfaction after meals.

2. Nutrient Absorption: Fats are necessary for the absorption of fat-soluble vitamins (A, D, E, and K) and other fat-soluble compounds. Consuming healthy fats alongside nutrient-rich foods allows your body to absorb and utilize these vital nutrients effectively.

3. Hormone Regulation: Fats are crucial for the production and balance of hormones in your body. Certain hormones, such as testosterone, estrogen, and cortisol, rely on fat for their synthesis. Including healthy fats in your diet supports hormonal balance and overall well-being.

4. Cell Structure and Protection: Fats are integral components of cell membranes, providing structural integrity and facilitating cell communication. They also help insulate and protect organs, maintain body temperature, and cushion joints.

Choose healthy sources of fats, such as monounsaturated fats found in avocados, nuts, and olive oil, and polyunsaturated fats from fatty fish, flaxseeds, and chia seeds. Limit saturated fats from animal sources and minimize trans fats found in processed and fried foods, as they can have negative health effects when consumed in excess.

Finding the right balance of carbohydrates and fats in your diet is individualized and depends on various factors like activity level, goals, and overall health. It's important to focus on quality, opting for complex carbohydrates and healthy fats, while moderating intake to align with your specific needs.

Remember, a well-rounded diet should include a balance of carbohydrates, fats, and proteins, along with an emphasis on whole, unprocessed foods.

Macro & Micronutrients - Summary

Macro and micronutrients are essential components of a healthy and balanced diet. Macronutrients, including carbohydrates, proteins, and fats, are needed in large quantities and provide energy and structural components to the body. Micronutrients, including vitamins and minerals, are required in smaller amounts and play vital roles in various bodily functions, including growth and development, immune system function, and energy production.

Carbohydrates are the body's primary source of energy, and they are found in various foods such as fruits, vegetables, grains, and dairy products. Proteins are essential for the growth and repair of tissues, and they are found in foods like meat, fish, eggs, beans, and nuts. Fats, while often maligned, are important for various bodily functions, including hormone production, insulation, and energy storage. They are found in foods like nuts, seeds, oils, and fatty fish.

Micronutrients, such as vitamins and minerals, play critical roles in the body's various systems, including immune function, bone health, and cognitive function. Some examples of micronutrients include iron, vitamin C, vitamin D, and calcium, which are found in foods such as leafy greens, citrus fruits, dairy products, and fortified foods.

While a balanced diet should include a variety of macronutrients and micronutrients, it's essential to remember that individual needs may vary depending on factors such as age, sex, and activity level.

How & Why You Should Track Your Daily Macros & Caloric Needs

A commonly asked question in training and nutrition is: should you track your daily calories and macros, and if so, how?

To answer that question we need to first address that it depends on your specific goals, lifestyle, and personal preferences. There are different approaches to nutrition in the fitness community, with some being very detailed and strict, while some just intuitively eating while trying to keep most of your foods healthy and non-processed.

I will break down 3 different individual types of nutritional tracking, with level 1 being the easiest and least precise type, and level 3 being the most thorough and precise.

Lvl 1: Intuitive eating approach: Intuitive eating is an approach to eating that involves tuning into your body's natural hunger and fullness cues to guide your food choices and eating habits. It's based on the idea that our bodies are equipped with an innate ability to regulate our food intake and maintain a healthy weight, as long as we listen to and trust our body's signals. The intuitive eating approach focuses on developing a healthy relationship with food and your body by prioritizing your physical and emotional needs. This approach involves permitting yourself to eat all types of food in moderation, without judgment or guilt. It also encourages paying attention to the sensory experience of eating, such as the taste, texture, and satisfaction level of the food. You base the food choices and portion sizes on your body's hunger signals, estimations of nutritional content, and your personal fitness goals.

Some key principles of intuitive eating include:

• Rejecting the diet mentality: This involves letting go of the idea that there is a "perfect" diet or weight and recognizing that restrictive dieting is often unnecessary and can be harmful to both physical and mental health.

• Making peace with food: This involves permitting yourself to eat all types of food in moderation, without labeling foods as "good" or "bad" and without feeling guilty or ashamed for enjoying certain foods.

• Honoring your hunger: This means tuning into your body's hunger signals and eating when you're hungry, rather than ignoring your hunger or eating out of habit or boredom.

• Respecting your fullness: This involves paying attention to your body's fullness signals and stopping eating when you're satisfied, rather than eating until you're overly full or uncomfortable.

There are 2 main situations where intuitive eating is going to be a good option:

1. If you've used intuitive eating until now and keep getting good results that you're satisfied with. That is why I mostly don't recommend this approach to complete beginners. Most of them will end up eating too much or too little. But for some people, it can work out just fine. If you're consistently progressing in your workouts and your weight and body fat percentage are moving in the right direction without counting your calories & macros, just continue with what you're doing and only switch to a more detailed system later on if your results stagnate (plateau).

1. If you're a skilled trainee who has obtained the necessary knowledge through practice. So, you've previously kept track of your macros, have a solid concept of what foods and portion sizes contain what, are aware of how your body reacts to different calorie intakes, and are aware of how to correctly modify your calorie and nutrient intake based on your degree of hunger.

Lvl 2: Tracking calories and only estimating your macros. This is simple enough to not have to revolve your entire day around your diet and also effective enough to get you near-optimal results. The total calorie intake is the most important part of your nutrition plan since that's what's going to dictate whether you gain, lose or maintain weight.

As long as your macronutrient intake is reasonably balanced, tracking total calories will usually be enough to get most if not all of the results. However, you need to keep the tracking precise. Don't forget to count the calories in sauces, beverages, etc.

Keep in mind that it's the average calorie intake over a few days that matter and not one specific day. Make sure your daily average for every week is in the range you want and that you're hitting your daily protein & fat minimums. I don't recommend doing a low-carb diet unless you have a specific reason for it, but protein and fat are the essential macronutrients you need to make sure you're getting enough of. Protein to build and repair muscle and fat to maintain optimal testosterone and other hormone levels. Make sure to get in at least 1.8 grams of protein per kilogram of body weight and at least 25% of your total calorie intake from fat.

Lvl 3: Full Macro & Calorie Tracking. You know precisely how many grams of protein, carbs, and fats you get in and the amount of calories you take in. This takes a lot of discipline and practice and will take a while to get consistent with hitting the same amounts of macros each day. There are 3 main situations where this applies:

1. You take training very seriously and you want to maximize every part of your results. Especially if you have to get in a certain shape until a certain deadline - e.g. a photo shoot, a physique competition, etc. Remember that tracking everything perfectly will only give you a small boost/improvement in the big picture. If that is worth it to you, then go ahead and do it.

1. You like it and knowing that you hit every macro and calorie precisely keeps you motivated. Most people find it unsustainable and too complicated, while some people prefer it.

1. You have never done it before. If you have never tracked calories and macros closely before, I recommend doing it for a temporary period to pick it up as an overall long-term skill. It's valuable in the long run even if you don't plan to do it as normal because you have a good understanding of which foods contain what and your body's needs, which makes it easier for you to effectively intuitively eat as well.

The people that *SHOULDN'T* do this are those with eating disorders or that are prone to them. You should also not do this if it causes you a lot of stress. If it messes with your social life and mental health, you shouldn't do this as a long-term thing.

In my experience and knowledge, most people are going to be better off moving towards an intuitive style of eating, and people who have tracked macros before will be able to do that better and easier. If you plan on tracking your daily caloric intake, you need to first figure out your daily caloric needs.

The number of calories you need to consume each day depends on several factors, including your age, gender, weight, height, activity level, and goals. Here's a detailed guide on how to calculate your daily caloric needs:

1. Determine your basal metabolic rate (BMR):

Your BMR is the number of calories your body burns at rest. This is the minimum number of calories your body needs to perform basic functions such as breathing, circulation, and maintaining body temperature. To calculate your BMR, you can use an online BMR calculator that takes into account your age, gender, weight, and height.

2. Calculate your total daily energy expenditure (TDEE):

Your TDEE is the total number of calories you burn in a day, including your BMR and any physical activity. To calculate your TDEE, you can multiply your BMR by an activity factor. The activity factor takes into account your activity level and ranges from sedentary (little or no exercise) to extremely active (intense exercise or sports). Here are the activity factors:

- Sedentary: BMR x 1.2

- Lightly active: BMR x 1.375

- Moderately active: BMR x 1.55

- Very active: BMR x 1.725

- Extremely active: BMR x 1.9

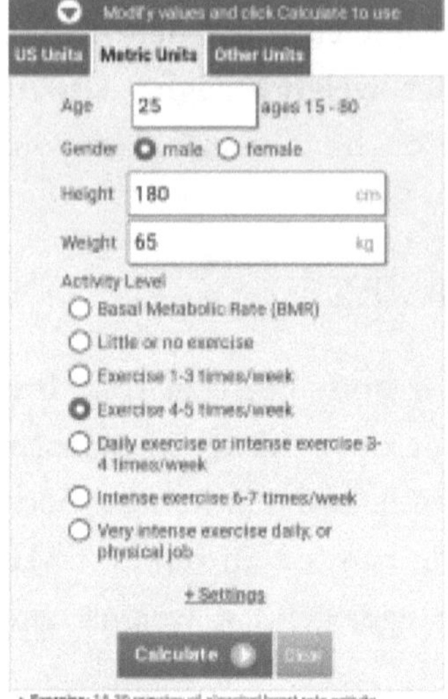

3. Determine your weight goal:

If your goal is to maintain your current weight, your daily caloric intake should be equal to your TDEE. If your goal is to lose weight, you will need to create a caloric deficit by consuming fewer calories than your TDEE. A calorie deficit of 500 calories per day is recommended for safe and sustainable weight loss. If you want to gain weight, you need to create a caloric surplus of around 300-500 calories to avoid excess fat gain.

4. Adjust your caloric intake based on your progress:

Once you have calculated your daily caloric needs, it's important to monitor your progress and adjust your caloric intake as needed. If you're not seeing the desired results, you may need to adjust your caloric intake or activity level. If you're losing weight too quickly, you may need to increase your caloric intake to prevent muscle loss and other negative effects.

If you decide that you want to track your macros as well, here's a guide and some information on how to do that:

1. Set your macronutrient goals: Before you can start tracking your macros, it's important to establish your specific macronutrient goals. This involves determining the ideal ratio of carbohydrates, proteins, and fats based on your individual needs, goals, and dietary preferences. You can consult a registered dietitian or use online calculators to help you determine your macronutrient targets.

However, you don't have to do any of these and if properly done you can just decide the ratio by yourself. As previously told, you should get at least 1.8 grams of protein per kilogram of body weight and get at least 25% of your total calorie intake from fat. The rest is totally up to you and won't matter much as long as you follow those 2 rules.

2. Choose a tracking method: There are several ways to track your macros, so choose a method that works best for you. Here are a few options:

a. Food diary/notebook: Use a notebook or a dedicated app to manually record the foods you consume throughout the day, along with their macronutrient content. You can find nutritional information on food labels or use online databases for accurate data.

b. Mobile apps: Utilize smartphone apps designed for macro tracking. These apps allow you to easily log your food intake, automatically calculate your macros, and provide a comprehensive overview of your progress.

c. Online platforms: Use online platforms that offer macro tracking features. These platforms often have extensive food databases, recipe calculators, and community support to help you stay on track.

3. Weigh and measure your food: To accurately track your macros, it's crucial to measure and weigh the foods you consume. Investing in a kitchen scale can be highly beneficial. Refer to food labels for accurate serving sizes, or use measuring cups and spoons when needed.

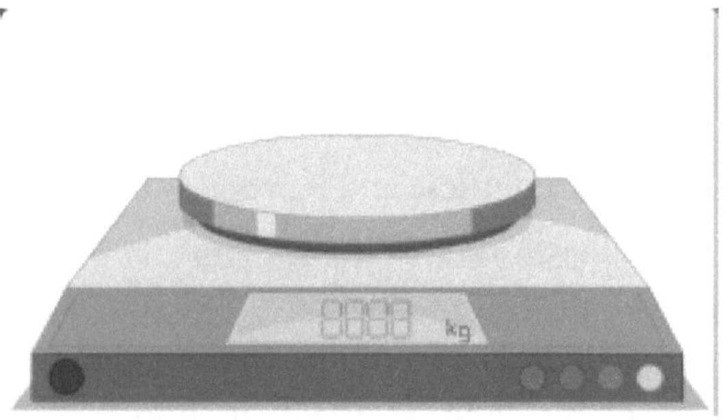

4. Record your meals and snacks: Log each meal and snack, including the specific foods, quantities, and cooking methods. Be as detailed as possible to ensure accurate tracking. Don't forget to account for beverages and condiments as well, as they can contribute to your overall macronutrient intake.

5. Stay consistent and be mindful: Consistency is key when tracking macros. Make it a habit to record your food intake consistently, ideally in real-time or shortly after each meal. This helps you stay accountable and provides an accurate representation of your daily macronutrient intake.

6. Adjust and evaluate: Regularly evaluate your progress and make adjustments as needed. If you're not seeing the desired results or experiencing any adverse effects, consider modifying your

macronutrient ratios or total calorie intake. Gradual adjustments can help you find the optimal balance for your goals.

Remember, tracking macros is a tool to help you achieve your dietary goals, but it's important to maintain a balanced and varied diet. Focus on consuming whole, nutrient-dense foods while considering your macronutrient targets. With consistent tracking and adjustments, you can better understand your eating habits and make informed choices to support your overall health and fitness goals.

Strategies for Creating a Sustainable & Effective Nutrition Plan for Fat-Loss

Creating a sustainable nutrition plan is essential for long-term success and overall well-being. It involves adopting healthy eating habits that are practical, flexible, and enjoyable, allowing you to nourish your body while maintaining a balanced lifestyle. Here are some strategies to help you develop a sustainable nutrition plan:

1. Set Realistic and Attainable Goals: Start by setting realistic and attainable nutrition goals that align with your individual needs and lifestyle. Avoid drastic or restrictive approaches that are difficult to sustain in the long run. Instead, focus on gradual changes and building healthy habits over time.

2. Emphasize Whole, Unprocessed Foods: Base your diet around whole, unprocessed foods that are rich in nutrients and minimally processed. These include fruits, vegetables, whole grains, lean proteins, legumes, nuts, and seeds. These foods provide essential vitamins, minerals, fiber, and antioxidants, promoting overall health and well-being.

3. Practice Portion Control: Pay attention to portion sizes to avoid overeating. Use visual cues, such as using smaller plates and bowls, to help regulate portion sizes. Listen to your body's hunger and fullness cues, and eat mindfully, savoring each bite. This allows you to enjoy your meals while maintaining control over your calorie intake.

4. Include a Variety of Food Groups: Aim to include a variety of food groups in your nutrition plan to ensure you receive a wide range of nutrients. Each food group offers unique health benefits, so aim for a colorful plate with a mix of fruits, vegetables, whole grains, lean proteins, and healthy fats.

5. Plan and Prepare Meals: Planning and preparing your meals in advance can help you make healthier choices and avoid relying on convenience foods. Set aside time each week to plan your meals, create a shopping list, and batch cook or meal prep. This allows you to have nutritious meals readily available, saving time and promoting healthier eating habits.

6. Practice Mindful Eating: Slow down and practice mindful eating. Pay attention to the sensory experience of eating, including the taste, texture, and aroma of your food. Eat without distractions, such as electronic devices, to fully appreciate and enjoy your meals. This helps you tune into your body's hunger and fullness signals, preventing overeating.

7. Honor Your Food Preferences: A sustainable nutrition plan should include foods you enjoy. Allow yourself flexibility and incorporate your favorite foods in moderation. Allowing occasional indulgences helps prevent feelings of deprivation and promotes a positive relationship with food.

8. Stay Hydrated: Proper hydration is vital for overall health and supports numerous bodily functions. Aim to drink adequate water throughout the day and limit sugary beverages. Carry a water bottle with you as a reminder to stay hydrated and consider flavoring your water with fruits or herbs to make it more enjoyable.

9. Seek Professional Guidance: Consider consulting with a registered dietitian or nutritionist who can provide personalized guidance and support. They can help you navigate your specific nutritional needs, address any concerns, and tailor a sustainable eating plan that works for you.

10. Practice Self-Care and Flexibility: Remember that sustainable nutrition goes beyond just the food you eat. Prioritize self-care, stress

management, and quality sleep, as these factors significantly impact your overall well-being. Be flexible and adaptable in your approach, allowing for life's unexpected changes while staying committed to your health goals.

Creating a sustainable nutrition plan is a lifelong journey. It's important to be patient, kind to yourself, and embrace progress over perfection. By incorporating these strategies into your daily life, you can develop a sustainable nutrition plan that supports your health, well-being, and long-term success.

Strategies for Creating a Sustainable & Effective Nutrition Plan for Weight Gain and Muscle Building

Creating a sustainable nutrition plan for weight gain and muscle building is crucial for achieving your goals while supporting your overall health and well-being. It involves providing your body with the right balance of nutrients and energy to promote muscle growth and recovery. Here are some strategies to help you develop a sustainable nutrition plan for weight gain and muscle building:

1. Set Caloric Surplus Goals: To gain weight and build muscle, you need to consume more calories than your body burns. Determine your daily caloric needs using online calculators or consult with a registered dietitian to estimate your requirements. Aim for a modest caloric surplus of around 250-500 calories per day to promote gradual weight and muscle gain while limiting fat gain.

2. Prioritize Protein Intake: Protein is essential for muscle growth and repair. Aim to consume an adequate amount of protein with each meal. The general guideline for individuals engaging in strength training is to consume around 0.8-1 gram of protein per pound of body weight. Include protein-rich foods such as lean meats, poultry, fish, eggs, dairy products, legumes, and plant-based protein sources like tofu and tempeh.

3. Consume Complex Carbohydrates: Carbohydrates provide the energy necessary for intense workouts and replenish glycogen stores. Focus on consuming complex carbohydrates, including whole grains, fruits, vegetables, and legumes. These sources provide essential nutrients, fiber, and sustained energy, supporting optimal

performance during workouts and promoting muscle glycogen replenishment.

4. Include Healthy Fats: Healthy fats provide additional calories (9 calories per gram, while protein and carbs contain 4 calories per gram) and support hormone production and overall health. Incorporate sources of healthy fats such as avocados, nuts, seeds, olive oil, and fatty fish like salmon. These fats also aid in nutrient absorption and help meet your daily caloric needs.

5. Eat Sufficiently Throughout the Day: To support muscle growth, aim to eat regular meals and snacks throughout the day. Include a combination of protein, carbohydrates, and fats in each meal to provide a balanced nutrient profile. Consider dividing your total caloric intake into smaller, frequent meals to ensure a consistent supply of nutrients and energy.

6. Hydrate Adequately: Proper hydration is crucial for overall health and optimal performance. Drink adequate water throughout the day to support digestion, nutrient absorption, and muscle function. Hydrate before, during, and after workouts to replace fluids lost through sweat. Remember, water is the main component of the body and represents approximately 76% of muscle mass.

7. Plan and Prepare Meals: Planning and preparing your meals in advance can help you stay on track with your nutrition plan. Set aside time each week to plan your meals, create a shopping list, and prepare nutritious meals and snacks. Having healthy options readily available will help you make better choices and avoid relying on processed or unhealthy foods.

8. Monitor Progress and Adjust as Needed: Regularly monitor your progress by tracking your weight, body measurements, and strength gains. Make adjustments to your nutrition plan based on your

results. If you're not seeing the desired weight gain or muscle growth, consider increasing your caloric intake slightly or adjusting your macronutrient ratios.

9. Practice Patience and Consistency: Building muscle and gaining weight takes time and consistency. Be patient with your progress and stay committed to your nutrition and workout plan. Consistency in your eating habits, combined with regular exercise and adequate rest, will yield the best results over the long term.

Remember, a sustainable nutrition plan for weight gain and muscle building should prioritize nutrient-dense foods, adequate caloric intake, and regular physical activity.

Meal Planning & Preparation

Meal planning is a powerful tool that can revolutionize your approach to nutrition and support your health and fitness goals. By taking a proactive approach to meal preparation and organization, you can ensure that you consistently nourish your body with the right foods, save time, and make healthier choices. Whether your goal is weight loss, muscle gain, or simply maintaining a balanced diet, meal planning can be your secret weapon.

One of the key benefits of meal planning is the ability to control your calorie intake and macronutrient balance. By carefully selecting and portioning your meals in advance, you can align them with your specific nutritional needs. This empowers you to make intentional choices that fuel your body optimally, promoting steady energy levels and supporting your desired body composition.

Additionally, meal planning helps you overcome the pitfalls of impulsive and unhealthy eating. When you have a clear plan in place, you're less likely to rely on convenience foods or succumb to unhealthy temptations. Instead, you can stock your kitchen with wholesome ingredients, ensuring that you always have nutritious options readily available.

Effective meal planning involves a few key steps. First, establish your goals and identify the specific dietary requirements that align with them. Consider factors such as calorie intake, macronutrient distribution, and any special dietary considerations you may have. Armed with this information, you can create a framework for your meal plan.

Next, focus on variety and balance. Include a wide range of nutrient-dense foods from all major food groups to ensure that you're meeting your body's needs for vitamins, minerals, and other essential nutrients. Aim for a colorful plate, incorporating a variety of fruits, vegetables, lean proteins, whole grains, and healthy fats.

Once you have your meals planned out, it's time to make a shopping list and hit the grocery store. Having a list helps you stay focused and avoid impulse purchases that may derail your meal plan. Choose fresh, high-quality ingredients whenever possible and be mindful of portion sizes to maintain balance and avoid waste.

With your ingredients in hand, set aside dedicated time for meal preparation. This may involve batch cooking, where you prepare larger quantities of certain foods that can be portioned and stored for later use. Invest in quality food storage containers to keep your meals fresh and easily accessible.

Remember that flexibility is key. Life can be unpredictable, and it's important to adapt your meal plan as needed. Allow room for occasional indulgences or spontaneous dining out while staying mindful of your overall nutrition goals.

Meal planning is a journey that requires some initial effort, but the rewards are well worth it. Not only does it support your health and fitness goals, but it also helps you develop a positive relationship with food and take control of your dietary choices.

Incorporate meal planning into your routine and experience the convenience, empowerment, and satisfaction it brings. From nourishing your body with wholesome meals to saving time and reducing stress, meal planning is a powerful strategy that can transform your eating habits and pave the way for a healthier, happier you.

Hydration

Proper hydration is essential for maintaining overall health and optimizing your fitness performance. When it comes to cardiovascular exercise for fat loss, staying hydrated becomes even more crucial. Adequate hydration supports various bodily functions and significantly impacts your energy levels, endurance, and the overall effectiveness of your workouts.

Staying hydrated during your journey offers several important benefits:

Enhanced Performance:

During exercise, dehydration can impair your performance, leading to fatigue, decreased endurance, and reduced exercise capacity. By staying properly hydrated, you can maintain optimal energy levels and perform at your best, maximizing the effectiveness of your workouts.

Temperature Regulation:

Training raises your body temperature and causes perspiration. Proper hydration helps regulate your body temperature, preventing overheating and ensuring efficient thermoregulation during your workouts.

Energy and Endurance:

Dehydration can negatively impact your energy levels and muscular endurance. When you're dehydrated, your body may struggle to deliver nutrients and oxygen to working muscles, resulting in fatigue and reduced exercise performance. By staying hydrated, you support proper blood flow, nutrient transport, and sustained energy levels throughout your workouts.

Appetite Control:

Adequate hydration can help regulate your appetite and contribute to your fat loss goals. Sometimes, thirst can be mistaken for hunger, leading to unnecessary snacking or overeating. By staying properly hydrated, you can better differentiate between thirst and hunger signals, promoting healthier eating habits and preventing unnecessary calorie consumption. However, hydration is also crucial for muscle building and preservation. The majority of your muscle tissue is water.

Practical Tips for Staying Hydrated:

- Drink sufficient water throughout the day, not just during workouts. Aim for a minimum of 8 cups (64 ounces) of water per day, adjusting intake based on individual needs and environmental conditions.

- Hydrate before starting your cardiovascular exercise. Consume around 16-20 ounces of water 2-3 hours before your workout and an additional 8-10 ounces 10-20 minutes before you begin.

- During longer-duration workouts, consider sipping on water or a sports drink that provides electrolytes to replenish fluids and essential minerals lost through sweating. Take small, regular sips to avoid discomfort during exercise.

- Rehydrate after your workouts to replenish fluids lost through sweat. Aim to drink 16-24 ounces of water or a recovery beverage within an hour of completing your workout.

- Monitor signs of dehydration, such as dark-colored urine, dry mouth, dizziness, or feelings of thirst. These indicators suggest the need to increase fluid intake.

Proper hydration is crucial in supporting your cardiovascular exercise routine for fat loss. By staying hydrated, you optimize your performance, sustain energy levels, regulate appetite, and enhance the effectiveness of your fat-burning workouts. Make hydration a priority by following these practical tips, ensuring you're adequately hydrated throughout the day and during your exercise sessions. Commit to maintaining optimal hydration levels, and you'll reap the benefits of improved fitness and successful fat loss and muscle gain results.

III: Resistance Training
The Benefits of Resistance Training for Muscle Building

Resistance training, also known as strength, hypertrophy training, or weightlifting, plays a crucial role in building muscle mass and achieving your fitness goals. It involves using external resistance, such as weights, cables, machines, or your own body weight/weighted body weight to challenge your muscles. Here are some key benefits of resistance training for muscle building:

1. Muscle Growth and Strength: Resistance training is highly effective in stimulating muscle growth and increasing muscular strength. When you subject your muscles to resistance, it causes microscopic damage to the muscle fibers. During the recovery process, the body repairs and rebuilds these fibers, resulting in muscle growth and increased strength. Regular resistance training with progressive overload—gradually increasing the intensity or resistance as you get stronger—promotes ongoing muscle development.

2. Increased Metabolic Rate: Building lean muscle mass through resistance training has a positive impact on your metabolic rate. Muscle tissue is metabolically active, meaning it requires more energy (calories) to maintain compared to fat tissue. As you gain muscle, your resting metabolic rate increases, leading to a higher calorie burn even at rest. This can support weight management goals and make it easier to maintain a healthy body composition.

3. Improved Body Composition: Resistance training helps to sculpt and shape your body by reducing body fat and increasing muscle size and definition. While cardiovascular exercise aids in burning

calories, resistance training helps to preserve and build muscle while promoting fat loss. This combination results in a more attractive and aesthetic physique.

4. Bone Health and Injury Prevention: Resistance training contributes to improved bone density and strength, reducing the risk of osteoporosis and fractures. The stress placed on the bones during resistance exercises stimulates bone remodeling, leading to stronger and denser bones. Additionally, resistance training strengthens the connective tissues, tendons, and ligaments, providing better joint stability and reducing the risk of injuries.

5. Enhanced Functional Strength: Resistance training improves functional strength, which translates into better performance in everyday activities and sports. Whether it's lifting heavy objects, climbing stairs, or participating in recreational activities, having a strong and functional musculoskeletal system allows you to perform tasks more efficiently and with a reduced risk of injury.

6. Hormonal Benefits: Resistance training can positively influence hormone levels in the body. It promotes the release of anabolic hormones such as testosterone and growth hormone, which are essential for muscle growth and repair, drive, motivation, health, and libido. These hormonal responses to resistance training contribute to muscle building and overall improvements in body composition.

7. Enhanced Mental Well-being: Engaging in resistance training not only benefits your physical health but also has positive effects on your mental well-being. Regular exercise, including resistance training, has been linked to reduced symptoms of depression and anxiety, improved mood, and increased self-confidence. The sense of accomplishment and progress achieved through resistance training can boost self-esteem and provide a positive outlook on overall

fitness and well-being. It can also give you confidence and a visually pleasing look to attract a potential mate.

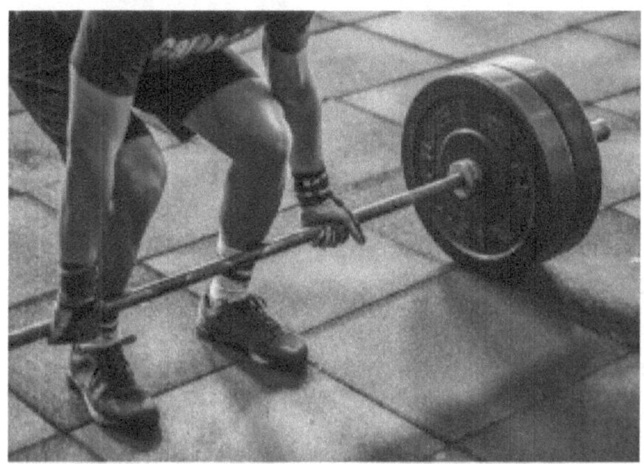

When incorporating resistance training into your fitness routine, it's important to prioritize proper form, progression, and recovery.

Remember that consistency is key when it comes to resistance training. Aim for at least two to three sessions per week *at minimum*, targeting different muscle groups, and allow for adequate rest and recovery between workouts. Over time, as you challenge your muscles progressively and follow a well-rounded nutrition plan, you can experience the remarkable benefits of resistance training for muscle building and overall fitness.

The Importance of Proper Technique and Form in Resistance Training

Proper technique and form are paramount when it comes to resistance training. Whether you're a beginner or an experienced lifter, paying close attention to how you perform exercises is crucial for maximizing results, preventing injuries, and ensuring long-term progress. Here are the key reasons why proper technique and form are of utmost importance:

1. Injury Prevention: One of the primary reasons to prioritize proper technique and form is to minimize the risk of injuries. Resistance training involves using external resistance, which can put stress on your muscles, joints, and connective tissues. Using an improper form, such as lifting too much weight or using momentum, can lead to strains, sprains, or more severe injuries. By maintaining proper alignment, controlling the movement, and engaging the correct muscles, you reduce the likelihood of accidents and enhance the safety of your workouts.

2. Targeted Muscle Engagement: Proper technique ensures that you're effectively targeting the desired muscle groups with each exercise. Different exercises have specific movement patterns and muscle activation requirements. By using proper form, you engage the intended muscles optimally, allowing for efficient muscle development and improved muscle symmetry. This is particularly important if you have specific goals, such as developing certain muscle groups or addressing muscular imbalances.

3. Maximizing Results: Performing exercises with proper form allows you to maximize the benefits of resistance training. By executing movements correctly, you enhance the quality of muscle contractions and stimulate muscle fibers more effectively. This can

lead to greater muscle activation, improved muscle recruitment, and ultimately better muscle growth and strength gains. Additionally, the proper form helps you maintain the intended range of motion, optimizing the exercise's effectiveness and ensuring you reap the desired training outcomes.

4. Building Strength and Progression: Proper technique and form facilitate a progressive overload approach, which is essential for strength development. Progressive overload involves gradually increasing the demands placed on your muscles to continue challenging them and promoting adaptation. By performing exercises with proper form, you can safely and effectively increase the weight or resistance over time, leading to continuous strength and muscle gains and improved performance.

5. Postural Alignment and Muscle Balance: Resistance training done with proper form can contribute to better postural alignment and muscle balance. Many people spend a significant portion of their day in positions that can lead to muscle imbalances and poor posture. By practicing exercises with proper technique, you strengthen the appropriate muscles, correct imbalances, and improve overall posture. This can alleviate muscle tension, reduce the risk of postural-related pain or injuries, and enhance overall functional movement patterns.

6. Mind-Muscle Connection: Focusing on proper technique and form cultivates a strong mind-muscle connection. Being aware of your body's movement and muscle engagement during each exercise helps you establish a deeper connection between your mind and the targeted muscles. This heightened awareness allows for more intentional and effective muscle contractions, leading to improved muscle control, coordination, and overall exercise performance. This also improves your muscle posing/flexing abilities.

To ensure proper technique and form during resistance training, consider the following tips:

1. Educate Yourself: Learn the correct form and technique for each exercise through reliable sources such as qualified fitness professionals, instructional videos, or reputable fitness resources. Take the time to understand the movement patterns, muscle groups involved, and key points of proper execution.

2. Start with Light Weights: Begin with lighter weights that allow you to focus on proper form and technique without compromising control or stability. Gradually increase the weight as you develop confidence and proficiency.

3. Prioritize Range of Motion and Avoid Ego Lifting: Perform exercises through their full range of motion, ensuring both the concentric (muscle shortening) and eccentric (muscle lengthening) phases are executed correctly. Avoid cutting corners or using excessive momentum.

4. Engage Stabilizing Muscles: Pay attention to the supporting muscles and stabilizers involved in each exercise. Strengthening these muscles helps maintain stability, joint alignment, and overall movement control.

5. Seek Guidance: Consider working with a certified personal trainer or strength and conditioning specialist who can provide personalized guidance, correct your form, and offer valuable feedback to optimize your workouts.

6. Practice Mindfulness: Approach each exercise with focus and intention. Visualize the targeted muscles working and concentrate on maintaining proper form throughout the entire set.

Remember, quality trumps quantity when it comes to resistance training. Prioritizing proper technique and form may mean lowering the weight or reducing the number of repetitions, but it will yield better long-term results and minimize the risk of injury. Embrace the mindset of continuous improvement and ensure that every rep counts. By doing so, you'll enhance the effectiveness of your workouts, maximize your progress, and enjoy the many benefits of resistance training.

The Role of Compound Exercises in Your Training Plan

Compound exercises play a fundamental role in any comprehensive training program, providing numerous benefits that contribute to overall strength, muscle development, and functional fitness. Unlike isolation exercises that target specific muscle groups, compound exercises involve multiple muscle groups and joints working together synergistically. Here's why incorporating compound exercises into your training program is crucial:

1. Efficient Use of Time: Compound exercises allow you to work multiple muscle groups simultaneously, making them highly time-efficient. Instead of dedicating separate exercises to target each muscle individually, compound movements engage larger muscle groups, maximizing your training efficiency and optimizing your time in the gym.

2. Muscle Development: Compound exercises stimulate significant muscle growth due to their ability to recruit multiple muscle groups. They provide a greater overall training stimulus compared to isolation exercises, leading to increased muscle fiber activation and growth. Compound movements such as squats, deadlifts, bench presses, and rows are excellent examples that engage major muscle groups, promoting overall muscular development.

3. Strength and Power: Compound exercises are highly effective for building strength and power. By involving multiple muscle groups, they allow you to lift heavier weights and exert greater force. As you progressively overload these movements, your strength and power levels will increase, translating into improved performance in various sports and physical activities.

4. Functional Movement Patterns: Compound exercises mimic natural, everyday movements and functional patterns. They promote better coordination, balance, and overall body control. By incorporating compound movements that involve pushing, pulling, squatting, and hinging, you enhance your ability to perform daily activities with greater ease and efficiency.

5. Core Activation and Stabilization: Compound exercises require the engagement of your core muscles to stabilize your spine and maintain proper posture throughout the movements. This results in improved core strength and stability, which are essential for overall strength, injury prevention, and optimal performance in other exercises and activities.

6. Hormonal Response: Compound exercises elicit a more significant hormonal response compared to isolation exercises. They stimulate the release of growth hormone and testosterone, which are crucial for muscle growth, fat loss, and overall body composition improvements. This hormonal response further enhances the effectiveness of your training program.

7. Caloric Expenditure: Due to their multi-joint nature and involvement of large muscle groups, compound exercises increase your caloric expenditure during and after your workouts. They elevate your heart rate, boost metabolism, and promote greater calorie burn. This makes compound movements beneficial for weight management, fat loss, and overall energy expenditure.

Here's a list of common compound exercises you can consider incorporating into your program:

1. Squats: Barbell squats, goblet squats, front squats, hack squats.

2. Deadlifts: Conventional deadlifts, sumo deadlifts, Romanian deadlifts.

3. Bench Press: Barbell bench press, dumbbell bench press, incline bench press.

4. Overhead Press: Barbell overhead press, dumbbell shoulder press, push press.

5. Rows: Barbell rows, dumbbell rows, seated cable rows, bent-over rows.

6. Pull-Ups/Chin-Ups: Wide grip pull-ups, close grip pull-ups, weighted pull-ups.

7. Lunges: Walking lunges, reverse lunges, stationary lunges.

8. Step-Ups: Dumbbell step-ups, and box step-ups.

9. Push-Ups: Standard push-ups, wide grip push-ups, decline push-ups, weighted push-ups.

10. Dips: Parallel bar dips, weighted dips.

11. Clean and Jerk: Olympic lift that involves explosiveness and full-body power.

12. Snatch: Olympic lift that targets multiple muscle groups and emphasizes power and speed.

13. Farmers Walk: Carrying heavy dumbbells or kettlebells for distance or time.

14. Kettlebell Swings: Full-body movement that combines a hip hinge and explosive movement.

15. Thrusters: Combining a front squat into an overhead press movement.

To incorporate compound exercises effectively into your training program, consider the following tips:

1. Prioritize Compound Movements: Make compound exercises the foundation of your workouts. Focus on incorporating movements such as squats, deadlifts, lunges, bench presses, overhead presses, rows, and pull-ups. These exercises provide the most bang for your buck in terms of muscle activation and overall development.

2. Progressively Overload: Gradually increase the weight or resistance used for compound exercises over time. This progressive overload principle challenges your muscles, stimulates growth, and helps you continually progress.

3. Ensure Proper Form: Technique and form are crucial for compound exercises. Master the correct form for each movement to optimize muscle activation, reduce the risk of injury, and maximize results. If needed, seek guidance from a qualified fitness professional to ensure proper execution.

4. Balance with Isolation Exercises: While compound exercises should form the core of your training, incorporating some isolation exercises can help target specific muscle groups and address any imbalances or weaknesses. Combine compound and isolation movements strategically to create a well-rounded training program.

5. Listen to Your Body: Pay attention to your body's feedback and adapt your training accordingly. If you experience any pain or discomfort during compound exercises, consult with a healthcare professional or fitness expert to address the issue and modify your training program if needed.

Incorporating compound exercises into your training program is essential for achieving a well-rounded and effective workout routine. By focusing on these multi-joint movements, you'll experience improvements in strength, muscle growth, functional fitness, and overall performance.

Isolation Exercises

While compound exercises take the spotlight in many training programs, isolation exercises also have an important role to play. Unlike compound movements that involve multiple muscle groups and joints, isolation exercises target specific muscles in isolation. Although they may not provide the same overall muscle activation as compound exercises, they offer unique benefits that can enhance your fitness journey. Here's why you should consider incorporating isolation exercises into your training program:

1. Muscle Targeting: Isolation exercises allow you to specifically target and isolate individual muscles or muscle groups. This level of precision can be beneficial for addressing specific weaknesses, imbalances, or lagging muscle groups. By focusing on a particular muscle, you can stimulate its development and improve overall muscle symmetry.

2. Muscle Definition and Detail: Isolation exercises can help enhance muscle definition and detail. By targeting specific muscles, you can stimulate greater hypertrophy and promote increased muscle separation and definition. This is particularly valuable for individuals looking to sculpt specific areas or achieve a more aesthetic physique.

3. Injury Rehabilitation and Prehabilitation: Isolation exercises can be useful for rehabilitating and strengthening specific muscles or joints following an injury. They allow you to focus on the injured area without placing excessive stress on surrounding muscles. Additionally, incorporating isolation exercises as part of your regular training routine can help prevent injuries by strengthening weak or vulnerable areas.

4. Mind-Muscle Connection: Isolation exercises provide an opportunity to develop a strong mind-muscle connection. By isolating specific muscles, you can develop a heightened awareness and control over their contraction. This connection can enhance your overall training performance and ensure optimal muscle activation during compound movements as well.

5. Variation and Muscle Stimulation: Adding isolation exercises to your training program introduces variety and new stimuli for your muscles. It can help break through plateaus and prevent training adaptation by providing different angles, ranges of motion, and resistance profiles. This can result in renewed muscle growth and improved overall muscle development.

When incorporating isolation exercises into your training program, consider the following tips:

1. Supplement Compound Movements: Isolation exercises should complement, not replace, compound exercises in your training program. Prioritize compound movements that engage multiple muscle groups and joints for overall strength and functional fitness. Use isolation exercises as supplementary movements to target specific muscles and provide better hypertrophy.

2. Proper Form and Technique: Just like with compound exercises, maintaining proper form and technique is crucial for isolation exercises. Focus on the mind-muscle connection, use controlled movements, and ensure a proper range of motion to maximize the effectiveness of each repetition.

3. Individual Goals and Needs: Select isolation exercises based on your individual goals and needs. Identify specific muscle groups that require additional attention and choose exercises that effectively target those areas. Consult with a fitness professional if you need

guidance in selecting the appropriate isolation exercises for your goals.

4. Balance and Prioritization: Strike a balance between compound and isolation exercises in your training program. Give priority to compound movements that provide overall strength and muscle development, while allocating appropriate time and energy to isolation exercises for targeted muscle work.

Some popular and effective isolation exercises are:

1. Bicep Curls: Targets the bicep muscle.

2. Tricep Extensions: Focuses on the triceps muscle.

3. Lateral Raises: Targets the lateral deltoid muscles of the shoulders.

4. Front raises: Targets the front deltoid muscles

5. Leg Curls: Isolates the hamstrings at the back of the thighs.

6. Leg Extensions: Targets the quadriceps muscles on the front of the thighs.

7. Calf Raises: Works the gastrocnemius and soleus muscles of the calves.

8. Cable Crunches: Focuses on the abdominal muscles for core strength.

Incorporating isolation exercises can bring diversity, precision, and targeted muscle development to your training program. By combining compound and isolation movements strategically, you can achieve a well-rounded, balanced approach to building strength, muscle, and overall fitness.

Strategies for Progressive Overload and Increasing Intensity

To continue making progress and achieving your fitness goals, incorporating strategies for progressive overload and increasing training intensity is essential. Progressive overload refers to gradually increasing the demands placed on your body during exercise to continually stimulate adaptations and improvements. Here are some effective strategies to implement progressive overload and increase training intensity:

1. Gradually Increase Resistance: One of the most straightforward and common ways to apply progressive overload is by increasing the resistance or weight you lift. As your strength improves, progressively add more weight to your exercises. This challenges your muscles and forces them to adapt and grow stronger over time.

2. Manipulate Repetitions and Sets: Adjusting the number of repetitions and sets you perform can help increase training intensity. As you become more proficient with an exercise, gradually increase the number of repetitions you complete. Additionally, you can add more sets to extend the overall volume of your workout. This increased workload challenges your muscles and promotes growth.

3. Adjust Rest Periods: Manipulating your rest periods between sets can significantly impact training intensity. Shortening the rest periods forces your muscles to work harder and recover more quickly. This can increase the metabolic stress placed on your muscles, leading to greater gains in strength and endurance. However, I don't recommend this if your goal is specifically muscle building and hypertrophy. The shorter your muscles rest, the less force they can exert, which means that you can miss out on potential muscle growth.

4. Vary Tempo and Speed: Another effective strategy is to manipulate the tempo or speed at which you perform exercises. Slowing down the eccentric (lowering) phase of a movement and focusing on controlled contractions increases time under tension, intensifying the stimulus on your muscles. Similarly, incorporating explosive movements and fast repetitions can enhance power and muscle fiber recruitment.

5. Incorporate Supersets and Compound Sets: Supersets and compound sets involve performing multiple exercises back-to-back without rest. This technique increases the workload and metabolic demand on your muscles, potentially stimulating greater muscle growth and improving overall conditioning. Combining exercises that target different muscle groups or movement patterns can provide an effective challenge.

6. Implement Progressive Training Techniques: Explore advanced training techniques to further enhance progressive overload. Techniques such as drop sets, pyramid sets, rest-pause training, and eccentric-focused training can help push your muscles to new limits and break through plateaus. These techniques introduce additional challenges and intensify your workouts.

7. Track and Monitor Progress: To effectively implement progressive overload, it's crucial to track and monitor your progress. Keep a workout log or use a fitness app to record your lifts, sets, and repetitions. This allows you to objectively assess your performance and ensure you're consistently increasing the demands placed on your body over time.

8. Periodize Your Training: Implementing a periodized training program can help systematically manage and optimize your training intensity. Periodization involves dividing your training into distinct phases, each with specific goals and intensity levels. It allows for

planned cycles of high and low-intensity periods, ensuring proper recovery and long-term progress.

Remember, progressive overload should be applied gradually and progressively over time. Avoid making sudden, drastic changes that may increase the risk of injury. Listen to your body, prioritize proper form and technique, and ensure adequate rest and recovery to support your training efforts. By incorporating these strategies, you can effectively apply progressive overload and continually increase the intensity of your workouts, leading to improved strength, muscle growth, and overall fitness.

Rep Ranges and Volume

When it comes to building muscle, understanding the principles of rep ranges and volume is essential. These factors play a significant role in determining the effectiveness of your workouts and the muscle-building stimulus you provide to your body. Here's a breakdown of rep ranges and volume and how they contribute to muscle growth:

Rep Ranges:

Rep ranges refer to the number of repetitions performed during an exercise set. Different rep ranges elicit varying physiological responses and adaptations in your muscles. Here are the commonly recognized rep ranges and their effects:

1. Low Rep Range (1-6 reps): This rep range primarily focuses on strength development. It allows you to lift heavier weights, recruit high-threshold motor units, and enhance neuromuscular efficiency. While the primary focus is on strength gains, it also contributes to muscle hypertrophy, especially when combined with higher-volume training.

2. Moderate Rep Range (7-12 reps): This rep range is often considered the sweet spot for muscle growth. It provides a balance between mechanical tension and metabolic stress. Moderate rep ranges stimulate muscle fibers effectively, promote hypertrophy, and increase muscular endurance. It's commonly used in traditional bodybuilding and strength training programs.

3. High Rep Range (12+ reps): This rep range primarily focuses on muscular endurance and metabolic stress. Higher reps target slow-twitch muscle fibers, enhance muscle endurance, and improve muscular conditioning.

Many individuals claim that the number of reps you perform doesn't matter as long as you train close to failure (0-3 reps within muscular failure). They argue that anywhere from 5 to 30 reps can stimulate the same amount of muscle growth. However, this perspective overlooks important factors that can impact the effectiveness of your workouts.

When you train with very high rep ranges, it becomes challenging to achieve true muscular failure. Instead, you may find yourself limited by factors such as cardiovascular stress, muscle burn, nausea, mental fatigue, and overall endurance. These effects tend to compound across multiple sets, shifting the focus of your workout towards conditioning and endurance rather than hypertrophy or strength development.

While it's perfectly fine to include some high-rep sets in your training routine, it's important to consider their placement. I recommend incorporating them closer to the end of your workout. This allows you to prioritize the heavier, lower rep ranges earlier in your session where you can focus on maximizing muscular strength and hypertrophy.

By strategically incorporating different rep ranges into your training program, you can target a variety of muscle fibers and stimulate overall muscle development.

Ultimately, finding the right balance between rep ranges is crucial. It's essential to challenge your muscles sufficiently without compromising proper form and execution. Listen to your body's feedback and adjust your training intensity accordingly. By incorporating a range of rep schemes and focusing on progressive overload, you can optimize your muscle-building potential and achieve your desired results.

Volume:

Volume refers to the total amount of work performed during a training session or over a specific period. It is typically calculated by multiplying the number of sets, reps, and weights lifted. Volume is a critical factor in muscle hypertrophy, as it provides a cumulative stimulus for growth. Here's how volume influences muscle development:

1. Set Volume: The number of sets performed for each exercise directly impacts muscle growth. Higher set volumes provide more opportunities for muscle fiber recruitment and stimulation. However, excessively high set volumes without adequate recovery can lead to overtraining, diminishing returns, and increased risk of injuries. Finding the right balance is crucial.

2. Total Volume: Total volume represents the overall workload of a training session or a specific training cycle. It takes into account the volume of all exercises performed. Progressive overload is key to building muscle, and gradually increasing total volume over time can help stimulate muscle growth. This can be achieved by adding more sets, increasing reps, or lifting heavier weights.

Strategies for Optimizing Muscle-Building Rep Ranges and Volume:

1. Periodization: Implement a periodization plan that incorporates different rep ranges and volume phases throughout your training program. This approach ensures sufficient variation and prevents plateaus.

2. Progressive Overload: Continually challenge your muscles by gradually increasing weight, reps, or sets over time. This progressive overload principle stimulates muscle growth and adaptation.

3. Individualization: Tailor your rep ranges and volume based on your fitness level, goals, and recovery capacity. Consider working with a qualified fitness professional to design a program that suits your specific needs.

4. Variation: Incorporate a variety of exercises, rep ranges, and training techniques to keep your muscles stimulated. This variation can also target different muscle fibers and promote well-rounded muscle development.

Junk Volume

In the world of fitness and strength training, the concept of junk volume has gained attention as a factor that can hinder progress and impede muscle growth. Junk volume refers to excessive training volume that does not contribute significantly to muscle stimulation or adaptation. It's the notion of "more is better" taken to an extreme, without considering the quality and effectiveness of the training stimulus.

Junk volume is exactly what it sounds like. Normal volume is the number of work/hard sets you do, and junk volume is garbage, worth nearly nothing.

Here's a closer look at junk volume and its implications:

1. Lack of Quality Stimulus: Junk volume typically involves performing excessive sets, reps, or exercises without a clear purpose or focus. It often leads to sacrificing proper form and execution in favor of quantity over quality. The result is a diminished ability to generate sufficient tension and overload on the muscles, hindering the potential for muscle growth.

2. Inefficient Use of Time and Energy: Engaging in excessive training volume without strategic planning can lead to wasted time and energy. Instead of allocating resources effectively to promote muscle development, junk volume spreads efforts too thin across various exercises or redundant movements. This can lead to suboptimal results and slower progress over time.

3. Increased Risk of Overtraining: Training with excessive volume without proper recovery can increase the risk of overtraining syndrome. Overtraining occurs when the body is subjected to excessive stress and insufficient time for recovery. This can lead to

decreased performance, stalled progress, increased fatigue, and heightened susceptibility to injuries.

4. Plateau in Progress: Engaging in junk volume can create a false sense of productivity, as individuals may feel they are putting in the work without seeing the desired results. However, without a focus on quality training stimulus and progressive overload, the body may adapt to the excessive volume without experiencing further gains in strength or muscle mass.

5. Quality over Quantity: The key to avoiding junk volume lies in prioritizing quality over quantity. Instead of mindlessly adding more sets or reps, focus on optimizing each repetition and maximizing the intensity of your workouts. Emphasize proper form, execute exercises with control and intention, and strive for progressive overload to elicit muscle adaptation.

6. Individualization and Programming: Every individual has unique training needs and capacities. Tailor your training volume based on your goals, recovery ability, and training experience. A well-designed program that incorporates appropriate volume, intensity, and rest intervals can maximize results while minimizing the risk of junk volume.

7. Listening to Your Body: Pay attention to the signals your body provides. If you consistently feel fatigued, lack motivation, or experience stagnation in progress despite high training volume, it may be a sign that you are engaging in junk volume. Adjust your training program accordingly, incorporating sufficient rest and recovery to allow for optimal muscle repair and growth.

Let's take a look at the 3 most common types of junk volume and how we can avoid them.

1. Excessive volume per workout: Let's say you're training your chest and after a warm-up, you grab a pair of dumbbells and do your first working set within 8-12 reps on the flat dumbbell press. This is a hard set and you finish within 1-2 reps of failure. Because the muscle is being shortened and lengthened under load with control, there is no doubt it will generate a high amount of mechanical tension within the pecs (chest). This set falls under what we call "effective volume".

If instead of one set you did 2 sets, both of these sets would be effective for stimulating muscle growth. And if you did 3 sets, it would be effective as well. But what if you did 10 sets? Would all of these 10 sets be equally effective and stimulate 10 times the growth, or would the stimulus per set eventually diminish to the point where we call them wasted sets?

It has been proven that the return per set will diminish, but at what point does it become junk? How many sets can you perform per workout until you're just wasting your time, energy, and ability to recover?

Studies have shown that up to around 6-8 working sets per muscle group per *workout*, you get pretty clear benefits in terms of muscle growth, but once you go above 6-8 sets you hit a pretty hard plateau and may even regress a little. However, this is different from how many weekly sets you need to generate maximum growth, which we will cover soon. Right now we are looking at how many sets we should do in a single workout instead.

Back to the chest example, yes, you could do sets beyond 6-8 e.g. 10, 14, or 20 sets in a single workout. However, those extra sets won't do much to grow your muscle and at a certain point will be counterproductive because now your chest will have a harder time recovering from all that volume. This doesn't refer to just one exercise but to the muscle working. So it doesn't matter if you do 10 sets of bench presses in one workout or 3 sets of push-ups, 3 sets of dumbbell presses, and 4 sets of chest presses. Some of those sets are most likely going to fall under the junk volume category.

If you feel like you need that much volume to keep progressing, you'd be better off splitting that volume out into separate workouts, or maybe you don't need as much volume as you think you do.

However, some of you reading this book might be genetic outliers and able to do more work without running into junk volume as easily. That's why you should use this information as a starting point and adjust the numbers up or down based on your progress and recovery. You need to also base your volume depending on how much you train until failure. If you push every set until absolute failure, your volume cap will be lower. Remember, even if you do fewer than 6 sets per workout that's fine as long as your total weekly set amount is sufficient.

From my experience, these numbers differ depending on the body part you're training. Some body parts tolerate and benefit from higher volume. For example, large muscles like the quads, glutes, or back seem to benefit from higher volumes, around 10-12 sets per workout.

1. Easy sets: This is the most common and the most pernicious type of junk volume there is, at least in commercial gyms and with casual lifters. Research shows that most lifters don't train hard enough to maximize muscle growth. In a study, people were asked to pick a weight they'd normally lift for 10 reps on the bench press and then the researchers had them lift it and get as many reps as they possibly could.

Only 22% of people got 10-12 reps (0-2 reps within failure), which is where you want to be if you want to maximize muscle growth.

31% got 13-15 reps (3-5 reps within failure), this will still build muscle, but if this is the majority of your routine you might have trouble getting past the newbie stage and progressively build muscle & strength over a long period. This technically isn't junk volume because it's still worth something, but it's not the optimal way to train for muscle growth.

47% of people got 16-20+ reps (6-10 reps within failure). This is junk volume and you'll never get past the intermediate stage by training this way. For optimal results, the majority of hypertrophy work should be within 0-3 reps from failure

1. Ultra-high-rep sets: Anything upwards of 40-50 reps and comparable to so-called easy sets, it isn't that ultra-high rep sets didn't do anything, they're just far from optimal. Another downside of ultra-high-rep work is that it creates a huge recovery demand for no added hypertrophic stimulus.

How Many Sets Per Week?

Now that we know how much volume is optimal in one workout per muscle group, it's time to address how much weekly volume is the best for hypertrophy as well.

Determining the optimal number of weekly sets per muscle group is a topic of great interest in the realm of hypertrophy training. While there is no one-size-fits-all answer, research and practical experience provide insights into the range that is typically effective for promoting muscle growth. Here's a closer look at the factors to consider and the general recommendations for optimal hypertrophy:

1. Individual Variations: Optimal training volume can vary depending on several factors, including individual genetics, training experience, recovery capacity, and overall lifestyle. Some individuals may respond better to higher training volumes, while others may require less volume to achieve optimal results. It's essential to listen to your body, monitor your progress, and make adjustments based on your response.

2. Range of Effective Volume: Research suggests that a weekly set range of approximately 10 to 20 sets per muscle group may be effective for promoting hypertrophy. This range is commonly used in resistance training programs and has shown positive results for many individuals. However, it's important to note that this is a general guideline, and individual responses may vary.

3. Spreading Volume Across Sessions: Distributing the weekly sets across multiple training sessions is a practical approach. For example, if you aim for 15 sets per week for a specific muscle group, you could split it into two sessions of 7 and 8 sets. Spreading the volume allows

for proper recovery between sessions and can help maintain training quality and intensity.

4. Progressive Overload and Adaptation: While training volume is an important factor, it's crucial to emphasize the principle of progressive overload. Increasing the number of sets without considering other variables, such as intensity and exercise selection, may not yield optimal results. Continually challenging your muscles with increasing loads, intensity techniques, and variations in exercises is key to triggering hypertrophy.

5. Listening to Your Body: As with any training program, it's important to listen to your body's feedback. Monitor your performance, recovery, and overall well-being. If you constantly struggle to recover or experience signs of overtraining, it may indicate that you're exceeding your optimal volume threshold. The same goes if you do a low amount of weekly sets and feel like your results stagnate, increase the weekly volume by a couple of sets. Adjusting your training volume accordingly can help prevent burnout and promote sustainable progress.

In general, you can get the majority of your gains potential with just 10 weekly sets per muscle group, and going up to 20 sets will get you some more gains, but it'd be slowly diminishing. Somewhere in the 10-20 sets per muscle group per week zone is probably the sweet spot for most people.

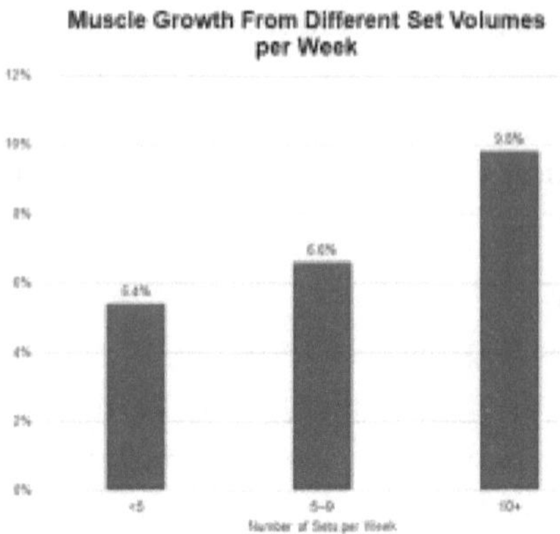

10 sets per week pushing close to failure is a minimum effective volume for a lot of people. Different people can respond differently to the same amount of work. If you consistently perform 20 or more weekly sets per muscle group pushing 0-3 reps within failure and you constantly feel fatigued, you aren't progressing, and you feel like you aren't recovering properly, you might need to do less.

Whereas if you're doing 10 sets per week close to failure and you feel like you aren't doing enough and you're not getting the results that you're looking for; you might need to do more.

However, this depends on the person that's training and we don't know the actual upper limit to how many weekly sets is "too much" and is counterproductive or junk. Even if you go up to 20-30 sets you can get significantly more gains than with 10 sets.

While there have been some studies that have shown a plateau in gains, there hasn't been a single study that shows a loss in muscle mass from increasing volume. This means we don't yet know where the limit is, whether it's 30, 40, or 50 sets isn't clear yet. Once again, this mostly depends on the individual training. But just because we haven't found an upper limit where volume becomes detrimental to muscle growth in the research, that isn't an endorsement for lifters (especially beginners) to do as much volume as possible.

It's also important to note that these volume marks are exercise specific. Some exercises will be more damaging and affect recovery more than others. A set of pull-ups may not count in the same way as a set of lat pull-downs. Volume isn't the only thing that matters, although it's very important.

Remember, finding the optimal number of sets per muscle group for hypertrophy is a process of experimentation and individualization. It's essential to consider your goals, recovery capacity, training experience, and overall lifestyle factors. Working with a qualified fitness professional can provide further guidance and help tailor your training program to your specific needs and goals.

Different Training Styles

1. Strength Training:

Strength training focuses on increasing maximal strength and is commonly associated with heavy resistance training. It involves lifting heavier weights for lower repetitions, typically in the range of 1-6 reps. The goal is to improve the body's ability to generate force and develop overall strength. Strength training often includes compound exercises like squats, deadlifts, bench presses, and overhead presses. It is often beneficial for athletes, e.g. fighters or runners.

2. Hypertrophy Training:

Hypertrophy training aims to stimulate muscle growth and increase muscle size. It involves moderate to high-volume training with moderate to heavy weights. The rep range commonly used is 6-12 reps, focusing on achieving muscle fatigue and metabolic stress. Hypertrophy training includes a variety of exercises targeting specific muscle groups and is often associated with bodybuilding.

3. Powerlifting:

Powerlifting is a competitive strength sport that focuses on three main lifts: squat, bench press, and deadlift. The goal is to lift as much weight as possible in these specific exercises. Powerlifters train for maximal strength and typically work with lower repetitions and heavier weights. The emphasis is on building total body strength and improving performance in the three lifts.

4. Calisthenics:

Calisthenics is a form of bodyweight training that uses one's body as resistance to build strength, endurance, and flexibility. It includes exercises such as push-ups, pull-ups, dips, squats, and various core exercises. Calisthenics training often incorporates elements of gymnastics, focusing on mastering bodyweight movements and progressing to more advanced exercises like muscle-ups, handstands, and human flags.

5. CrossFit:

CrossFit is a high-intensity training program that combines elements of strength training, cardiovascular conditioning, and functional movements. It incorporates a wide range of exercises and workouts, including weightlifting, gymnastics, cardiovascular exercises, and bodyweight movements. CrossFit aims to develop overall fitness, including strength, endurance, agility, and power.

6. Circuit Training:

Circuit training involves performing a series of exercises in a specific sequence with minimal rest in between. It combines resistance training and cardiovascular exercises, targeting multiple muscle groups and providing a full-body workout. Circuit training can be customized to focus on strength, endurance, or both, depending on the exercises and intensity used.

7. High-Intensity Interval Training (HIIT):

HIIT involves alternating between periods of high-intensity exercises and short rest or recovery periods. It is a time-efficient training style that combines cardiovascular exercises with bursts of intense effort. HIIT workouts can vary in duration and intensity, but they typically last between 10-30 minutes. It is effective for improving cardiovascular fitness, burning calories, and boosting metabolism.

8. Functional Training:

Functional training focuses on exercises that mimic everyday movements or activities. It aims to improve strength, stability, flexibility, and coordination to enhance overall functionality and performance in daily life or specific sports. Functional training often includes exercises using free weights, resistance bands, stability balls, and bodyweight movements that engage multiple muscle groups simultaneously.

9. Olympic Weightlifting:

Olympic weightlifting is a sport that includes two main lifts: the snatch and the clean and jerk. It requires explosive power, strength, and technique to lift maximal weights overhead. Olympic weightlifting training focuses on developing power, speed, and coordination through specific exercises and variations of the snatch and clean and jerk.

Each training style has its unique benefits and objectives. The choice of training style depends on individual goals, preferences, and available resources. Many individuals incorporate elements from multiple training styles to create a well-rounded fitness routine that addresses various aspects of strength, endurance, flexibility, and overall fitness. It's important to seek proper guidance and gradually progress in any training style to ensure safety and maximize results. Hypertrophy training is the best option for people who seek to build muscle and achieve an aesthetic, attractive body while being strong & healthy as well.

Different Training Splits

1. Full Body Split:

The full-body split involves working out the entire body in each training session. It typically includes compound exercises that target multiple muscle groups. This split is suitable for beginners or individuals with limited time for training, as it allows for frequency and stimulus to all major muscle groups in each session.

2. Bro Split:

The bro split, also known as the body part split, involves dedicating each training day to a specific muscle group. For example, chest on Monday, back on Tuesday, legs on Wednesday, and so on. This split is popular among bodybuilders and advanced lifters who aim to target individual muscle groups with high volume and intensity. It allows for greater focus on specific muscle groups but may result in longer recovery times for each muscle group, which is one of the reasons why this split isn't optimal for natural lifters.

3. Push Pull Legs (PPL) Split:

The push-pull legs split divides training sessions into three main categories: push exercises (chest, shoulders, triceps), pull exercises (back, biceps), and leg exercises. This split allows for balanced training and efficient recovery as different muscle groups are targeted on different days. It is a popular choice for individuals looking to optimize training volume while still allowing adequate rest and recovery.

4. Upper/Lower Split:

The upper/lower split involves dividing training days into upper-body and lower-body workouts. Upper body days typically target the chest, back, shoulders, and arms, while lower body days focus on the legs and core. This split allows for higher frequency and volume for each muscle group compared to a bro split while still providing adequate rest and recovery.

5. Push/Pull/Legs Split:

The push-pull-legs (PPL) split is a training program that categorizes exercises into push, pull, and leg movements. Every separate day contains either push, pull, or leg exercises. Push exercises target pushing muscles, pull exercises target pulling muscles, and leg exercises focus on lower body training. It offers balanced muscle development and customization options for individual goals. It can range from 3 up to 6 training days a week.

6. Hybrid Splits:

Hybrid splits combine different training methods and principles. Examples include combining elements of full-body workouts with isolated exercises or alternating between strength-focused and hypertrophy-focused sessions. Hybrid splits can be customized to fit an individual's specific goals, preferences, and time availability.

When choosing a training split, consider your goals, training experience, schedule, and recovery capacity. It's important to strike a balance between providing adequate stimulus to each muscle group and allowing sufficient recovery for optimal progress.

Remember, there is no one-size-fits-all approach to training splits, and what works for one person may not work for another. Experimentation and listening to your body's feedback are key to finding the split that suits your individual needs and helps you achieve your fitness goals. Consulting with a qualified fitness professional can provide further guidance and assistance in selecting the most appropriate training split for you.

The Most Effective Training Split For Building Muscle

When it comes to building muscle and stimulating hypertrophy, which type of split you choose isn't going to play much of a role. As long as you're training hard consistently, sleeping enough, eating enough, and training with proper form you will build an incredible body.

However, some splits generally suit people who want to build muscle better than other splits. The most popular splits for building muscle are:

1. Bro split
2. Push Pull Legs Split
3. Upper lower split
4. Full body split

Let's look at the pros and cons of each of these and see which one suits the best for you:

1. Bro split

Pros:

1. Targeted Focus: The bro split allows for dedicated focus on individual muscle groups during each session. This can be appealing for individuals looking to prioritize specific areas for muscle growth.

2. High Volume and Intensity: The bro split often incorporates higher volume and intensity, as each muscle group is trained intensely once per week. This can stimulate muscle hypertrophy and provide a challenging workout experience.

3. Recovery Time: With a week-long training cycle, the bro split provides ample time for rest and recovery for each muscle group. This can be beneficial for individuals who require more time between sessions to recover and rebuild muscle.

4. Variation and Flexibility: The bro split allows for flexibility in exercise selection and variation, which can help prevent boredom and keep motivation high. It also allows for customization to target specific muscle groups based on individual goals.

Cons:

1. Lower Training Frequency: One of the main drawbacks of the bro split is its lower training frequency for each muscle group. Since each muscle group is typically trained once per week, this may not optimize the potential for muscle growth compared to higher-frequency training splits because having all your weekly sets for a muscle group in one workout isn't the best option for muscle building.

2. Potential Imbalances: Without careful planning, the bro split may lead to muscle imbalances if certain muscle groups are neglected or not given adequate attention. This can result in uneven development and potential injury risk.

3. Limited Skill Development: The bro split may not be ideal for individuals seeking to improve specific skills or performance in activities such as sports or athletic endeavors. It primarily focuses on muscle hypertrophy rather than overall functional fitness.

4. Time Commitment: The bro split typically requires a significant time commitment, as each training session may involve targeting one or two muscle groups with multiple exercises. This may not be feasible for individuals with limited time availability.

5. Potential Plateaus: Over time, the bro split may lead to training plateaus, as the training frequency and volume are limited.

It's important to consider these pros and cons when deciding if the bro split is the right approach for you. It may be suitable for individuals who enjoy a targeted focus on specific muscle groups and prioritize intensity in their training. However, for optimal muscle growth and overall fitness, incorporating elements of higher frequency and overall body training may be beneficial.

2. Push-Pull-Legs (PPL) Split:

Pros:

- Allows for dedicated focus on specific muscle groups during each session.

- Provides adequate recovery time for each muscle group.

- Allows for high volume and frequency of training.

- Can be easily modified and customized based on individual needs.

- Offers variation and versatility in exercise selection.

Cons:

- Requires careful planning to ensure balanced muscle development.

- Difficult to emphasize weak points because of multiple muscle groups trained in one day

3. Upper-Lower Split:

Pros:

- Allows for higher training frequency for each muscle group.

- Balances upper and lower body training.

- Provides ample recovery time between sessions.

- Allows for flexibility in organizing training days and rest days.

Cons:

- May require longer workout sessions to accommodate both upper and lower body exercises.

- May result in higher central nervous system (CNS) fatigue due to increased frequency.

- May require more planning and coordination for exercise selection and progression.

4. Full-Body Split:

Pros:

- Allows for high training frequency for each muscle group.

- Suitable for individuals with limited time availability or beginners (it builds a strong foundation for newbies).

- Can be effective for overall strength development.

- Allows for efficient use of compound exercises.

Cons:

- May require longer workout sessions due to training the entire body in each session.

- May lead to higher overall fatigue and require careful management of intensity and volume.

- May limit the focus on specific muscle groups during each session.

- May be less suitable for advanced lifters seeking more targeted muscle development.

So, which split is *the best* for hypertrophy and building muscle? Let's dive even deeper into that.

Training with the bro split consistently with proper form, good nutrition, and while pushing close to failure on each set you can definitely make good progress and build an amazing physique. However, due to its low training frequency (once a week per muscle group) and a variety of other factors, it's inferior to the other splits (at least for natural lifters).

When volume is matched, training each muscle at least 2 times per week results in significantly greater muscle growth than training each muscle just once a week. This means that even if you have the same weekly volume for a muscle, splitting that volume into different workouts rather than just one leads to better results.

It's likely due to higher training frequencies allowing your body to:

- Optimize protein synthesis response throughout the week

- Enable you to perform higher-quality sets because of less fatigue

- Avoid junk volume

For example, if you perform 20 sets for your back per week by training with the bro split, you'd have to perform 5 exercises with 4 sets each in just one workout. You'd start fatiguing after your first set and your performance would decrease from then on.

If you instead split those sets into 2 separate workouts, you'd fatigue less and perform your sets with better quality since you're not doing it all at once. This would lead to better muscle stimulus and potentially more muscle growth.

Now moving forward and knowing that the bro split isn't the best out of these 4 splits, which one is the best for you, upper lower, push-pull, or full body?

All of these splits are great and stimulate almost completely equal amounts of muscle growth. However, based on my training and coaching experiences, the progress of many lifters seems to diminish quicker with the upper lower and full body splits than with the Push Pull Legs rest and repeat (6 training days a week) split. Another effective and advanced training split is: Push, Pull, Legs, Rest, Upper, Lower (5 training days per week). These splits allow you to spread your training volume into different workouts and not have to stay in the gym for hours (like with the upper lower or full body splits) which means you're less likely to have junk volume in your routine.

It's important to consider your personal preferences, schedule, recovery capacity, and individual goals when selecting a training split. Experimenting with different approaches and monitoring your progress will help you determine which training split works best for you. Remember, adherence to the program and consistent effort are key factors in achieving hypertrophy goals regardless of the chosen split.

Building Your Training Plan

Congratulations on taking the first step toward achieving your fitness goals! Building an effective training plan is essential for maximizing your progress, whether you aim to build muscle, increase strength, or improve overall fitness. In this chapter, we will guide you through the process of creating a training plan that is tailored to your individual needs, preferences, and goals. By understanding the key components and principles of a well-structured training program, you will be equipped with the knowledge to design a plan that optimizes your results and keeps you motivated on your fitness journey.

1. Assessing Your Goals and Current Fitness Level:

- Clarifying Your Goals: Begin by clearly defining your fitness goals. Do you want to build muscle, lose fat, increase strength, improve cardiovascular fitness, or a combination?

- Evaluating Your Current Fitness Level: Assess your current fitness level to determine your starting point. This includes factors such as strength, endurance, flexibility, and overall fitness.

2. Determining Training Frequency:

- Understanding Training Frequency: Decide how many days per week you can commit to training. Consider factors like time availability, recovery capacity, and other commitments.

- Balancing Frequency and Recovery: Find a balance between training frequency and allowing enough time for recovery and muscle adaptation.

3. Selecting the Right Training Split:

- Exploring Different Training Splits: Understand the various training splits, such as full-body, upper-lower, push-pull-legs, and bro splits. Consider your preferences, goals, and available time when choosing the most suitable split for you.

- Balancing Muscle Group Emphasis: Ensure that your training split allows for balanced development of all major muscle groups to avoid imbalances and injury risks.

4. Structuring Exercise Selection:

- Incorporating Compound Exercises: Prioritize compound exercises that target multiple muscle groups simultaneously, such as squats, deadlifts, bench presses, and rows. These exercises provide a solid foundation for strength and muscle growth.

- Adding Isolation Exercises: Include isolation exercises to target specific muscles and address any weaknesses or imbalances and make your physique more defined and aesthetic. Examples include bicep curls, tricep extensions, and lateral raises.

5. Manipulating Training Variables:

- Progressive Overload: Understand the importance of progressively increasing the demands placed on your muscles over time. Continually challenge yourself by increasing weight, repetitions, or intensity to stimulate muscle growth and strength gains.

- Volume and Intensity: Manipulate training volume (sets and repetitions) and intensity (load or effort) to create appropriate stimuli for muscle adaptation.

- Periodization: Consider implementing periodization strategies, such as alternating between phases of higher volume and intensity, to prevent plateaus and maintain long-term progress.

6. Tracking Progress and Adjustments:

- Monitoring Your Progress: Keep track of your workouts, including exercises, sets, repetitions, and weights used. Measure your progress regularly to assess improvements and identify areas for adjustment.

- Adjusting Your Plan: Modify your training plan periodically based on your progress, changing goals, and individual preferences. Adapt the program to prevent stagnation and ensure continued progress.

7. The Warm-Up and Cool-Down:

The warm-up and cool-down are crucial components of a training plan. The warm-up prepares your body for exercise, reducing the risk of injury and enhancing performance. The cool-down promotes recovery and flexibility, aiding in muscle relaxation and preventing post-workout stiffness.

Warm-Up:

1. Injury Prevention: Reduces the risk of injury by preparing muscles and joints.

2. Enhanced Performance: Improves muscle activation and range of motion.

3. Mental Preparation: Helps transition to a focused mindset.

Components: Cardiovascular activity, dynamic stretching, and exercise-specific warm-up sets (e.g., bench press).

Cool-Down:

1. Recovery and Injury Prevention: Removes waste products and reduces muscle soreness.

2. Promotes Flexibility: Improves muscle and joint flexibility.

3. Mental Relaxation: Unwinds and reduces stress.

Components: Low-intensity exercise, static stretching, foam rolling, or self-massage.

The Cool-Down isn't mandatory, but if you have the time to do it, I recommend it.

Incorporating these principles optimizes your workout experience, prevents injuries, and promotes overall well-being.

By following these steps and principles, you can build an effective and personalized training plan that aligns with your goals and maximizes your results. Remember, consistency, proper form, and gradual progression are key.

Now that you know the key components and principles of making a good training plan, it's time to list the best exercises for each muscle group and show how to actually structure and put together your training plan.

Considering you have already chosen the split you'll train by, training frequency, and other factors, let's see how an effective workout plan can look.

Let's start with the Full Body 3-day split:

The Full Body 3-Day Training Split

A full-body 3-day training split is an effective way to work all major muscle groups while allowing sufficient rest and recovery between sessions. Here's how you can structure your training split and select exercises for each day:

Day 1:

1. Compound Lower Body Exercise: Start with a compound movement such as squats or lunges to target your quadriceps, hamstrings, and glutes. These exercises engage multiple muscle groups and build overall lower body strength. Also don't forget to add a calf raise variation, either seated, machine, Smith machine, or any other variation.

2. Upper Body Push: Perform exercises like bench presses or push-ups to target your chest, shoulders, and triceps. This helps develop upper body pressing strength and muscle definition.

3. Upper Body Pull: Include exercises like pull-ups or rows to target your back and biceps. These movements build upper-body pulling strength and promote a balanced physique.

4. Core Exercise: Incorporate a core exercise like planks or crunches to strengthen your abdominal muscles and improve core stability.

5. Optional Isolation Exercises: If time permits, you can add some isolation exercises like bicep curls or lateral raises to further target specific muscle groups.

Day 2:

1. Compound Upper Body Exercise: Start with a compound movement such as an overhead press or dumbbell row to target your shoulders, back, and arms.

2. Lower Body Exercise: Perform exercises like deadlifts or hip thrusts to target your posterior chain, including your glutes, hamstrings, and lower back. Add some kind of calf-raising variation as well. These movements build lower body strength and enhance overall athleticism.

3. Pushing Exercise: Include exercises like bench presses or dumbbell shoulder presses to target your chest, shoulders, and triceps.

4. Pulling Exercise: Incorporate exercises like pull-ups or lat pulldowns to target your back and biceps. These movements build upper-body pulling strength and promote a balanced physique.

5. Core Exercise: Add a core exercise of your choice to strengthen your abdominal muscles and improve core stability.

Day 3:

1. Compound Lower Body Exercise: Start with a compound movement such as squats or lunges to target your quadriceps, hamstrings, and glutes. Add a calf raise variation. These exercises engage multiple muscle groups and build overall lower body strength.

2. Upper Body Push: Perform exercises like bench press or overhead press to target your chest, shoulders, and triceps. This helps develop upper body pressing strength and muscle definition.

3. Upper Body Pull: Include exercises like pull-ups or rows to target your back and biceps. These movements build upper-body pulling strength and promote a balanced physique.

4. Core Exercise: Incorporate a core exercise like planks or cable crunches to strengthen your abdominal muscles and improve core stability.

5. Optional Isolation Exercises: If time permits, you can add some isolation exercises like bicep curls or lateral raises to further target specific muscle groups.

Ideally, with a 3-day full-body training split you should workout every other day, e.g. Monday, Wednesday, and Friday.

Now, let's take a look at how this can look as a workout template:

Day 1: Full Body

Warm-Up:

- Cycling: 5 minutes (or any other optional cardiovascular activity)

- Squats: 3-5 sets of 8-15 reps (gradually increase the weight)

Workout:

1. Squats: 3 sets of 8-12 reps
2. Bench Press: 3 sets of 8-12 reps
3. Incline Dumbbell Press: 3 sets of 8-12 reps
4. Bent-Over Rows: 3 sets of 8-12 reps
5. Seated Dumbbell Overhead Press: 3 sets of 8-12
6. Romanian Deadlifts: 3 sets of 8-12 reps
7. Pull Ups: 3 sets of 6-12 reps
8. Hanging Leg Raises: 3 sets of 8-15 reps
9. Standing Barbell Calf Raises: 3 sets of 8-12 reps

Cool-Down:

- Light Cycling: 5-10 minutes

- Static Stretches 30 sec each (e.g., chest stretch, quad stretch)

Day 2: Full Body

Warm-Up:

- Jogging: 5 minutes (or any other optional cardiovascular activity)

- Deadlifts: 3 sets of 8-15 reps

Workout:

1. Deadlifts: 3 sets of 6-12 reps
2. Bulgarian Split Squats (uni-lateral): 3 sets of 8-12 reps
3. Seated Cable Row: 3 sets of 6-12 reps
4. Chest Press Machine: 3 sets of 8-12 reps
5. Lat Pulldowns: 3 sets of 8-12 reps
6. Seated Shoulder Press (Machine): 3 sets of 8-12 reps
7. Lateral Raises: 3 sets of 8-12
8. Seated Calf Raises: 4 sets of 6-15

Cool-Down:

- Walking/Light Jogging: 5-10 Minutes

- Optional Static Full Body Stretches: 30 sec each position

Day 3: Full Body

Warm-Up:

- Leg Swings: 15 reps for each leg

- Squats: 3 sets of 10 reps

Workout:

1. Squats: 3 sets of 8-12 reps

2. Bench Press : 3 sets of 8-12 reps
3. Chest Supported Dumbbell Row: 3 sets of 8-12 reps
4. Cable Chest Fly: 3 sets of 8-12 reps
5. Leg Extension: 3 sets of 8-12 reps
6. Seated Leg Curl: 3 sets of 8-12 reps
7. Pull Ups: 3 sets of 8-12 res
8. Lateral Raises: 3 sets of 8-12 reps
9. Standing Barbell Calf Raises: 3 sets of 8-15 reps

Cool-Down:

- Calf Stretch: 30 sec

- Chest Stretch: 30 sec

- Tricep stretch: 30 sec

- Lat stretch: 30 sec

- Hamstring stretch: 30 sec

- Quad stretch: 30 sec

Keep in mind that this is just one example of a full-body 3-day training split. You can customize the exercises and order based on your preferences and needs. It's always beneficial to seek guidance from a qualified fitness professional to ensure proper form and technique.

Now, let's do this with the Upper/Lower 4-day split

The upper body sessions should include pulling and pushing movements that train the muscles of the back, arms, chest, shoulders, etc.

During the lower body sessions, you should incorporate squatting variations, leg curl variations, calf raise variations, and other exercises that load the leg muscles. Toward the end of the session, you can include some core/abdominal work.

As a template, it can look like this:

Day 1: Upper Body

Warm-up:

- 5-10 minutes of light cardio (e.g., brisk walking, cycling, or rowing)

- Bench Press: 3 Warm Up sets

Workout:

1. Bench Press: 3 sets of 8-12 reps

2. Seated Cable Rows: 3 sets of 8-12 reps

3. Chest Press Machine: 3 sets of 6-15 reps

4. Overhead Press: 3 sets of 8-12 reps

5. Lat Pulldowns: 3 sets of 8-12 reps

6. Dumbbell Bicep Curls: 3 sets of 10-15 reps

7. Tricep Dips: 3 sets of 10-15 reps

8. Lateral Raises: 3 sets of 8-15 reps

Cool-down:

- 5-10 minutes of low-intensity cardio (e.g., walking or light cycling)

- Static stretches for the upper body (e.g., chest stretch, tricep stretch)

Day 2: Lower Body

Warm-up:

- 5-10 minutes of light cardio (e.g., brisk walking, cycling, or rowing)

- Dynamic stretches for the lower body (e.g., leg swings, walking lunges)

Workout:

1. Squats: 3 sets of 8-12 reps

2. Romanian Deadlifts: 3 sets of 8-12 reps

3. Stationary Lunges: 3 sets of 10-15 reps per leg

4. Calf Raises: 4 sets of 12-15 reps

5. Leg Extensions: 3 sets of 8-15 reps

6. Hanging Leg Raises: 3 sets of 10-15 reps

Cool-down:

- 5-10 minutes of low-intensity cardio (e.g., walking or light cycling)

- Static stretches for the lower body (e.g., hamstring stretch, quad stretch)

Day 3: Rest

Day 4: Upper Body

Warm-up:

- 5-10 minutes of light cardio (e.g., brisk walking, cycling, or rowing)

- Incline Dumbbell Press: 3 warm-up sets

Workout:

1. Incline Dumbbell Press: 3 sets of 8-12 reps

2. Chest Supported Dumbbell Rows: 3 sets of 8-12 reps

3. Cable Fly: 3 sets of 10-15 reps

4. Shoulder Press Machine: 3 sets of 8-12 reps

5. Pull-Ups: 3 sets of 8-12 reps

6. Cable Face Pulls: 3 sets of 8-12 reps

7. Hammer Curls: 3 sets of 10-15 reps

8. Tricep Pushdowns: 3 sets of 10-15 reps

9. Lateral Raises: 3 sets of 8-15 reps

Cool-down:

- 5-10 minutes of low-intensity cardio (e.g., walking or light cycling)

- Static stretches for the upper body (e.g., chest stretch, tricep stretch)

Day 5: Lower Body

Warm-up:

- 5-10 minutes of light cardio (e.g., brisk walking, cycling, or rowing)

- Deadlifts: 3 warm-up sets

Workout:

1. Deadlifts: 3 sets of 8-12 reps

2. Leg Press: 3 sets of 8-12 reps

3. Bulgarian Split Squats: 3 sets of 10-15 reps per leg

4. Seated Calf Raises: 3 sets of 12-15 reps

5. Hack Squats: 3 sets of 8-15 reps

6. Hanging Leg Raises: 3 sets of 10-15 reps

Cool-down:

- 5-10 minutes of low-intensity cardio (e.g., walking or light cycling)

- Static stretches for the lower body (e.g., hamstring stretch, quad stretch)

Day 6-7: Rest

Now, let's do the same with the Push/Pull/Legs 6-day split:

Day 1: Push (Chest, Shoulders, Triceps)

Warm-up:

- 5-10 minutes of light cardio (e.g., brisk walking, cycling, or rowing)

- Barbell Bench Press: 3 warm-up sets

Workout:

1. Barbell Bench Press: 3 sets of 8-12 reps

2. Dumbbell Shoulder Press: 3 sets of 8-12 reps

3. Incline Dumbbell Fly: 3 sets of 10-15 reps

4. Tricep Dips: 3 sets of 10-15 reps

5. Cable Lateral Raises: 3 sets of 10-15 reps

6. Skull Crushers: 3 sets of 10-15 reps

Cool-down:

- 5-10 minutes of low-intensity cardio (e.g., walking or light cycling)

- Static stretches for the upper body (e.g., chest stretch, tricep stretch)

Day 2: Pull (Back, Biceps)

Warm-up:

- 5-10 minutes of light cardio (e.g., brisk walking, cycling, or rowing)

- Deadlifts: 3 warm-up sets

Workout:

1. Deadlifts: 3 sets of 8-12 reps

2. Lat Pulldowns: 3 sets of 8-12 reps

3. Barbell Rows: 3 sets of 8-12 reps

4. Hammer Curls: 3 sets of 10-15 reps

5. Seated Cable Rows: 3 sets of 10-15 reps

6. Preacher Curls: 3 sets of 10-15 reps

7. Barbell Shrugs: 3 sets of 8-15 reps

Cool-down:

- 5-10 minutes of low-intensity cardio (e.g., walking or light cycling)

- Static stretches for the upper body (e.g., back stretch, bicep stretch)

Day 3: Legs (Quadriceps, Hamstrings, Glutes, Calves)

Warm-up:

- 5-10 minutes of light cardio (e.g., brisk walking, cycling, or rowing)

- Walking Lunges: 3 sets of 10-15

Workout:

1. Squats: 3 sets of 8-12 reps

2. Leg Press: 3 sets of 8-12 reps

3. Romanian Deadlifts: 3 sets of 8-12 reps

4. Walking Lunges: 3 sets of 10-15 reps per leg

5. Leg Extensions: 3 sets of 10-15 reps

6. Standing Calf Raises: 3 sets of 12-15 reps

Cool-down:

- 5-10 minutes of low-intensity cardio (e.g., walking or light cycling)

- Static stretches for the lower body (e.g., hamstring stretch, quad stretch)

Day 4: Rest

Day 5: Push (Chest, Shoulders, Triceps)

Warm-up:

- 5-10 minutes of light cardio (e.g., brisk walking, cycling, or rowing)

- Incline Dumbbell Press: 3 warm-up sets

Workout:

1. Incline Dumbbell Press: 3 sets of 8-12 reps

2. Chest Press Machine: 3 sets of 8-12 reps

3. Dumbbell Chest Fly: 3 sets of 10-15 reps

4. Tricep Pushdowns: 3 sets of 10-15 reps

5. Lateral Raises: 3 sets of 10-15 reps

6. Skull Crushers: 3 sets of 10-15 reps

Cool-down:

- 5-10 minutes of low-intensity cardio (e.g., walking or light cycling)

- Static stretches for the upper body (e.g., chest stretch, tricep stretch)

Day 6: Pull (Back, Biceps)

Warm-up:

- 5-10 minutes of light cardio (e.g., brisk walking, cycling, or rowing)

- Banded Pull-Ups

Workout:

1. Pull-Ups: 3 sets of 8-12 reps

2. Seated Cable Row: 3 sets of 8-12 reps

3. Single-Arm Dumbbell Rows: 3 sets of 8-12 reps per arm

4. Hammer Curls: 3 sets of 10-15 reps

5. Cable Face Pulls: 3 sets of 10-15 reps

6. Concentration Curls: 3 sets of 10-15 reps

Cool-down:

- 5-10 minutes of low-intensity cardio (e.g., walking or light cycling)

- Static stretches for the upper body (e.g., back stretch, bicep stretch)

Day 7: Legs (Quadriceps, Hamstrings, Glutes, Calves)

Warm-up:

- 5-10 minutes of light cardio (e.g., brisk walking, cycling, or rowing)

- Smith Machine Squats: 3 warm-up sets

Workout:

1. Smith Machine Squats: 3 sets of 8-12 reps

2. Bulgarian Split Squats: 3 sets of 8-12 reps per leg

3. Romanian Deadlifts: 3 sets of 8-12 reps

4. Leg Extensions: 3 sets of 10-15 reps

5. Leg Curls: 3 sets of 10-15 reps

6. Seated Calf Raises: 3 sets of 12-15 reps

Cool-down:

- 5-10 minutes of low-intensity cardio (e.g., walking or light cycling)

- Static stretches for the lower body (e.g., hamstring stretch, quad stretch)

And lastly, you can adjust the split to whatever your preference is. You can do a Push/Pull/Legs/Upper/Lower 5-day split, Push/Pull/Legs/Full Body, etc.

Remember to adjust the weights and reps based on your fitness level and goals, and listen to your body to ensure proper form and technique.

Perform each exercise with proper form and technique. Use weights that challenge you (ideally 0-2 reps within failure) within the given rep range.

You can make amazing progress regardless of which split you choose. The split you select will only provide a slight difference in the muscle you gain and the fat you lose. The key is to pick the split that suits you the most, you like the most, and aligns with your circumstances and goals.

It's always recommended to consult with a qualified fitness professional to personalize your workout plan and ensure it aligns with your abilities and circumstances.

Resting Between Sets

Resting between sets is a crucial aspect of hypertrophy training that often goes overlooked. The appropriate rest periods can significantly impact your ability to maximize muscle growth and performance during your workouts. When aiming for hypertrophy with a rep range of 0-3 reps within failure, it's important to consider the following factors when determining your rest intervals:

1. Recovery: When training with heavy weights and moderate reps, your muscles and central nervous system require adequate time to recover. The rest period allows your muscles to replenish their energy stores and removes metabolic waste products, helping to reduce fatigue and optimize performance.

2. ATP Replenishment: Adenosine triphosphate (ATP) is the primary energy source for intense muscular contractions. During rest periods, ATP stores can be replenished, ensuring you have sufficient energy for the next set. Longer rest periods allow for more complete ATP restoration.

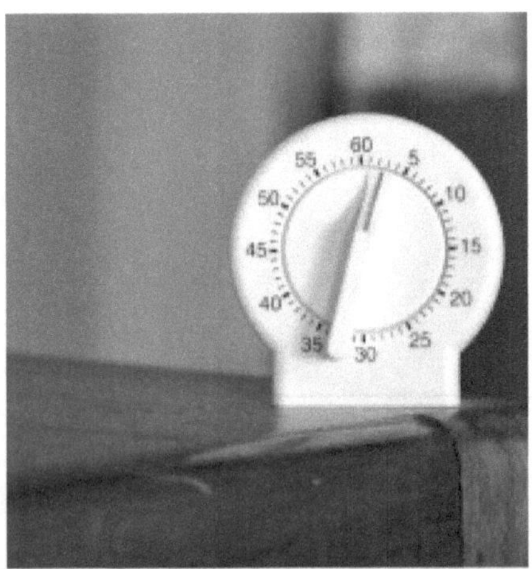

3. Training Intensity: Resting for the appropriate duration between sets allows you to maintain a high level of training intensity. This ensures that each set is performed with proper form and maximum effort, leading to optimal muscle stimulation and growth.

4. Oxygenation: Adequate rest periods allow for proper oxygenation of the working muscles. Oxygen plays a vital role in energy production and helps prevent the accumulation of metabolic byproducts such as lactic acid. Sufficient oxygenation during rest helps minimize fatigue and enables better performance on subsequent sets.

Considering these factors, a recommended rest period for hypertrophy training with moderate reps (0-3 reps within failure) is typically around 2-3 minutes between sets. This duration allows for sufficient recovery, ATP replenishment, and oxygenation while maintaining a high level of training intensity. However, it's important to note that individual preferences and conditioning levels may vary. Some individuals may find that they require slightly shorter or longer rest periods to optimize their performance and recovery.

Remember, rest periods are not set in stone and can be adjusted based on your individual needs, workout goals, and the specific exercises you're performing. Listen to your body, pay attention to your performance and fatigue levels, and make adjustments accordingly. It's always beneficial to experiment and find the rest periods that work best for you while still challenging yourself and promoting progress in your training.

List of Exercises

Here's a list of 5-10 great exercises for each major muscle group, you can pick a couple of these and include them in your training plan:

Chest:

1. Bench Press Variations (Incline, Flat, Barbell, Dumbbell, Smith Machine, etc.)

2. Machine Chest Press

3. Seated Cable Press

4. Cable Crossovers

5. Dumbbell Fly

Back:

1. Deadlifts

2. Pull-Ups/Chin-Ups

3. Barbell Rows

4. Lat Pulldowns

5. Seated Cable Rows

Shoulders:

1. Overhead Press (Barbell or Dumbbell)

2. Machine Shoulder Press

3. Lateral Raises

4. Rear Delt Dumbbell Fly

5. Face Pulls

Biceps:

1. Barbell Curls

2. Dumbbell Curls

3. Hammer Curls

4. Preacher Curls

5. Concentration Curls

6. Cable Curls

7. Incline Dumbbell Curls

8. EZ Bar Curls

9. Spider Curls

10. Chin-Ups

Triceps:

1. Dips

2. Close Grip Bench Press

3. Skull Crushers

4. Tricep Pushdowns

5. Overhead Tricep Extension

6. Diamond Push-Ups

Legs (Quadriceps, Hamstrings, Glutes):

1. Squats (Barbell, Dumbbell, or Smith Machine)

2. Lunges (Walking or Stationary)

3. Deadlifts (Conventional or Sumo)

4. Leg Press

5. Leg Extensions

6. Leg Curls

7. Bulgarian Split Squats

8. Hip Thrusts

9. Sissy squats

10. Hack Squats

Abdominals:

1. Planks (Standard or Variations)

2. Cable Crunches

3. Hanging Leg/Knee Raises

4. Bicycle Crunches

5. Woodchoppers

6. Ab Rollouts

These exercises are highly effective for targeting the respective muscle groups. However, it's important to note that individual preferences, fitness levels, and available equipment may vary. There are lots of other great exercises for each of these muscle groups.

It's always beneficial to consult with a qualified fitness professional to tailor the exercises to your specific needs and goals, ensuring proper form and technique.

Should You Train When Sick?

A common question in the fitness community is: Should You Train When Sick? Let's answer this from a scientific perspective.

First off, I have to say that if you're contagious, stay home and out of the gym for the sake of other members.

What if you have a private gym or you're not contagious? Should you train when sick?

First, assess the severity of the sickness: If you have severe symptoms like chest congestion, high fever, or difficulty breathing, it's best to avoid exercise altogether and focus on getting better. However, if you have mild symptoms like a runny nose, headache, or slight fatigue, you can train. A general rule is: if it's neck or above, you can train. Below the neck and you should skip training. So if you have mild symptoms, you have to make a decision yourself by making a cost-benefit analysis.

Assuming you're not using your sickness as an excuse to skip working out, it takes 2-4 weeks to see significant losses in muscle size and strength. Even if you take that much time off of training, you will get back to your previous state fairly quickly because of muscle memory. A full week off due to sickness is very unlikely to negatively affect your long-term progress.

If you're unsure whether you are using your sickness as an excuse, go to the gym and do some light/moderate intensity cardio. This will help you see and feel if you are in a good position to train or not. If after 10-15 minutes of light to moderate cardio you still feel lightheaded or not ready to get a good gym session in, leave it at that and go home. There's no risk in doing this since cardio will benefit you if you're sick anyway.

If you take time off and notice your physique appears smaller or flatter, it is most likely due to glycogen loss, not actual muscle loss (atrophy). Glycogen and hydration levels will return to normal very quickly as soon as you begin to refuel and rehydrate again.

In summary:

- If you're contagious, stay out of public gyms

- Light cardio will benefit you if you're sick

- Up to 3 weeks of not working out is unlikely to ruin your long-term progress

- Any muscle size loss in that period is most likely just glycogen and water loss and can be regained quickly.

IV: Cardio & HIIT for Fat Loss
The Benefits of Cardiovascular Exercise

Cardiovascular exercise, commonly referred to as cardio, plays a crucial role in fat loss and overall weight management. While resistance training is essential for building muscle and increasing metabolic rate, incorporating cardiovascular exercise into your fitness routine can significantly enhance your fat-loss efforts and give you numerous health benefits.

Cardiovascular exercise involves engaging in activities that elevate your heart rate and increase your breathing rate for an extended period. This includes activities like running, cycling, swimming, brisk walking, and various aerobic workouts. When performed consistently and with appropriate intensity, cardiovascular exercise can yield several benefits for fat loss:

1. Caloric Expenditure: Cardiovascular exercise helps burn calories, contributing to a calorie deficit necessary for fat loss. By engaging in cardio, you increase your energy expenditure, helping create an overall calorie deficit when combined with a balanced diet.

2. Enhanced Metabolic Rate: Regular cardiovascular exercise can boost your metabolism both during and after your workout. It increases the number of calories your body burns at rest, known as the resting metabolic rate, which supports fat loss by increasing overall energy expenditure.

3. Fat Utilization: Cardiovascular exercise stimulates the body to use stored fat as a fuel source. As you engage in aerobic activities, your body taps into fat stores to provide energy, aiding in fat loss over time.

4. Improved Cardiovascular Health: Cardiovascular exercise strengthens your heart and improves overall cardiovascular health. It enhances your heart's ability to pump blood efficiently, improves circulation, and reduces the risk of heart disease and other related conditions.

5. Stress Reduction: Regular cardio sessions can help alleviate stress and promote mental well-being. It releases endorphins, also known as "feel-good" hormones, which can improve mood, reduce anxiety, and support overall mental health.

When incorporating cardiovascular exercise into your fat loss regimen, consider the following guidelines:

1. Frequency: Aim for at least 150 minutes of moderate-intensity cardio or 75 minutes of vigorous-intensity cardio per week, spread across multiple sessions.

2. Intensity: Find a balance between a moderate and vigorous intensity that challenges your cardiovascular system. It should elevate your heart rate, make you breathe harder, and induce a sweat. Gradually increase intensity over time to continually challenge your body.

3. Duration: Start with shorter sessions and gradually increase the duration as your fitness level improves. Aim for 30 to 60 minutes per session, depending on your fitness goals and time availability.

4. Variety: Incorporate different forms of cardiovascular exercise to prevent monotony and keep your workouts enjoyable. Mix activities like running, cycling, swimming, and group fitness classes to engage different muscle groups and prevent plateaus.

5. Progression: Continually challenge yourself by increasing the intensity, duration, or frequency of your cardio sessions. This helps

avoid adaptation and ensures ongoing fat loss and fitness improvements.

Remember to listen to your body, stay hydrated, and choose activities that you enjoy. It's important to consult with a healthcare professional before starting any new exercise program if you have any underlying health concerns.

Cardiovascular exercise is an essential component of an effective fat-loss strategy. When combined with proper nutrition and resistance training, it can help you achieve your weight loss goals, improve overall fitness, and promote a healthy lifestyle. Cardio should be done by everyone because of its huge positive impact on our health, not only those who want to lose weight.

The Benefits of High-Intensity Interval Training (HIIT)

High-Intensity Interval Training (HIIT) has gained immense popularity in the fitness world due to its time efficiency and impressive health benefits. This exercise approach involves alternating short bursts of intense exercise with brief recovery periods. The unique intensity and structure of HIIT workouts offer numerous advantages that can help you achieve your fitness goals and improve your overall well-being.

Efficient Fat Burning:

One of the primary benefits of HIIT is its ability to maximize fat burning in a shorter time frame. The intense bursts of exercise elevate your heart rate and stimulate your metabolism, leading to an increased calorie burn during and even after your workout. HIIT has been shown to enhance both aerobic and anaerobic fitness, making it an effective strategy for reducing body fat and improving body composition.

Time-Saving:

For those with busy schedules, HIIT is a time-saving exercise option. Traditional steady-state cardio workouts typically require longer durations to achieve similar results. With HIIT, you can achieve substantial cardiovascular and metabolic benefits in as little as 15 to 30 minutes. This time efficiency makes HIIT an excellent choice for individuals seeking effective workouts that can be easily incorporated into their daily routines.

Increased Cardiovascular Fitness:

HIIT workouts challenge your cardiovascular system by pushing your heart rate to higher levels. The intense intervals followed by short recovery periods improve your cardiovascular capacity and oxygen utilization. Regular HIIT training can lead to enhanced heart health, improved endurance, and increased aerobic fitness levels.

Muscle Preservation and Strength:

Contrary to common belief, HIIT can be beneficial for muscle preservation and even muscle growth. HIIT may not be the most effective workout routine to build lean muscle mass. HIIT, however, can help preserve or retain lean muscle mass. The intense nature of HIIT workouts triggers muscle fiber recruitment, stimulating muscle preservation/development. Additionally, the metabolic demands of HIIT workouts can help preserve lean muscle mass while promoting fat loss. This is particularly valuable for individuals aiming to improve their body composition by reducing fat while maintaining or increasing muscle size.

Metabolic Benefits:

HIIT has been shown to have positive effects on insulin sensitivity, glucose metabolism, and fat oxidation. Regular HIIT training can improve insulin sensitivity, leading to better blood sugar control and reduced risk of type 2 diabetes. Moreover, HIIT workouts have been associated with increased post-workout calorie expenditure, which can support weight management and metabolic health.

Adaptability and Variety:

HIIT offers versatility and can be adapted to various fitness levels and preferences. You can incorporate a wide range of exercises into HIIT routines, including bodyweight exercises, cardio activities, and strength training movements. This flexibility allows you to customize your workouts based on personal preferences, fitness goals, and equipment availability.

High-Intensity Interval Training (HIIT) is a powerful training method that offers numerous benefits for individuals seeking efficient workouts and significant fitness improvements. From efficient fat-burning and time-saving advantages to cardiovascular fitness enhancements and metabolic benefits, HIIT has proven to be an effective and versatile exercise approach. Incorporating HIIT workouts into your fitness routine can help you achieve your goals, whether it's improving body composition, boosting cardiovascular health, or increasing overall fitness levels.

Strategies for Incorporating Cardio and HIIT into Your Training Program

1. Determine Your Goals:

Before incorporating cardio and HIIT into your training program, it's crucial to identify your specific goals. Are you aiming to improve cardiovascular fitness, burn fat, enhance athletic performance, or maintain overall health? Understanding your objectives will guide your approach and help you select the most appropriate cardio and HIIT exercises.

2. Select Suitable Cardio Activities:

Cardio exercises come in various forms, such as running, cycling, swimming, rowing, and dancing. Choose activities that you enjoy and that align with your fitness level, goals, and preferences. Aim for a mix of low-impact and high-impact cardio workouts to diversify your training routine. Incorporate steady-state cardio sessions for longer-duration endurance training and HIIT sessions for intense bursts of effort.

3. Integrate HIIT Workouts:

HIIT involves short bursts of high-intensity exercise alternated with periods of rest or low-intensity recovery. These workouts are time-efficient and effective for boosting metabolism, burning calories, and improving cardiovascular fitness. Include HIIT sessions two to three times per week, focusing on exercises like sprints, burpees, jumping jacks, or kettlebell swings. Adjust the work-to-rest ratio based on your fitness level and gradually increase the intensity and duration as you progress.

4. Plan for Proper Recovery:

Intense cardio and HIIT workouts place significant demands on your body. Allow sufficient time for recovery between sessions to prevent overtraining and reduce the risk of injuries. Incorporate active recovery days with lighter cardio exercises or low-impact activities like walking or yoga. Prioritize quality sleep, adequate nutrition, and hydration to support your recovery process and optimize your training results.

5. Implement Progressive Overload:

Similar to strength training, progressive overload is essential in cardio and HIIT workouts. Gradually increase the intensity, duration, or frequency of your workouts to challenge your body and promote continuous adaptation. You can progress by increasing the speed, resistance, or incline of your cardio exercises, or by modifying the work-to-rest ratios in your HIIT sessions. Monitor your progress, listen to your body, and make adjustments accordingly.

6. Combine Cardio and Resistance Training:

To create a well-rounded training program, integrate both cardio and resistance training. Resistance exercises help build strength, promote muscle growth, and enhance overall performance. Alternate between cardio and resistance training days or consider combining the two. This approach allows you to enjoy the benefits of both training modalities and achieve a balanced fitness routine.

7. Keep It Varied and Enjoyable:

Avoid monotony by incorporating a variety of cardio exercises and HIIT workouts into your training program. Experiment with different training modalities, try new workout formats, and explore outdoor activities. Keeping your workouts varied and enjoyable will not only prevent boredom but also promote long-term adherence to your fitness routine.

Tailoring your cardio and HIIT workouts to your specific goals is essential for optimizing your training program. Here are some key considerations for different objectives:

1. Fat loss and weight management: If your primary goal is to shed body fat and manage weight, there are a few strategies you can employ with cardio and HIIT:

- High-intensity interval training (HIIT): Incorporate HIIT workouts into your routine as they are highly effective for fat loss. Focus on short bursts of intense exercise followed by brief recovery periods. This helps elevate your heart rate, increase calorie burn, and stimulate fat metabolism. If you do resistance training and cardio/ HIIT on the same day, do the cardio/HIIT after you've finished resistance training.

- Longer duration steady-state cardio: Include longer cardio sessions at a moderate intensity, such as jogging or cycling, for extended periods (e.g., 45-60 minutes). This helps create a calorie deficit and promotes fat utilization as an energy source.

- Time under tension: Opt for longer intervals during HIIT sessions, such as 30-60 seconds of work followed by shorter recovery periods. This helps increase overall training volume and calorie expenditure.

- Combine cardio with resistance training: Incorporate workouts that combine cardio exercises with resistance training. This can boost calorie burn during and after the workout while promoting muscle maintenance or growth.

2. Cardiovascular fitness and endurance: If improving cardiovascular health and endurance is your primary focus, consider the following strategies:

- Steady-state cardio: Engage in longer duration cardio sessions at a moderate intensity. This helps improve cardiovascular efficiency and endurance by challenging the aerobic energy system.

- Progressive overload: Gradually increase the duration or intensity of your cardio workouts over time to continue challenging your cardiovascular system and promote adaptations.

- Interval training: Incorporate longer intervals of higher intensity efforts into your cardio sessions. For example, alternate between a moderate pace and a faster pace for specific time intervals (e.g., 2 minutes moderate, 1 minute fast).

- Tempo runs: Include tempo runs, which involve maintaining a comfortably hard pace for an extended period. This helps improve lactate threshold and aerobic capacity.

3. Performance and athletic conditioning: If you're an athlete or focused on improving performance, consider these strategies:

- Specificity: Choose cardio exercises that mimic the movements and demands of your sport or activity. For example, sprint intervals for a sprinter, agility drills for a soccer player, or heavy-bag drills if you're a fighter.

- Sport-specific intervals: Incorporate intervals that replicate the energy demands of your sport. For instance, short, intense bursts of effort followed by brief recovery periods for sports requiring quick bursts of power.

- Cross-training: Include a variety of cardio exercises to develop well-rounded fitness. This can enhance overall conditioning and help prevent overuse injuries.

- Periodization: Implement periodization in your training program, alternating between different phases of intensity and volume to optimize performance and prevent plateaus.

These strategies are just general guidelines, and it's important to personalize your approach based on your fitness level, preferences, and any specific considerations or limitations you may have. It's also beneficial to seek guidance from a qualified fitness professional who can provide further insights and tailor your training program to your goals.

By tailoring your cardio and HIIT workouts to your goals, you can maximize the effectiveness of your training program and achieve the desired outcomes more efficiently. Stay consistent, listen to your body, and enjoy the journey as you work towards your fitness aspirations.

V: Recovery and Rest

Adequate sleep is a crucial factor for both muscle building and fat loss. Let's explore the importance of sleep concerning these goals:

1. Muscle Building:

- Hormonal balance: During sleep, your body releases important hormones like growth hormone (GH) and testosterone, which play a key role in muscle repair, recovery, and growth. Insufficient sleep can disrupt hormonal balance, hindering muscle-building processes.

- Protein synthesis: Sleep promotes protein synthesis, the process by which your body builds and repairs muscle tissue. It allows for the optimal utilization of dietary protein to support muscle recovery and growth.

- Muscle recovery: Sleep is a period of rest and recovery for your muscles. It helps repair muscle damage caused by intense exercise and reduces muscle soreness. Sufficient sleep ensures your muscles are ready for subsequent workouts.

- Energy restoration: Sleep replenishes glycogen stores in your muscles, providing them with the necessary energy for intense workouts. With ample energy, you can perform better during training sessions, leading to more effective muscle-building exercises.

2. Fat Loss:

- Metabolism and energy balance: Sleep plays a role in regulating metabolism and energy balance. Inadequate sleep can disrupt these processes, leading to imbalances in appetite-regulating hormones, such as ghrelin and leptin. This can increase hunger and cravings, making it more challenging to maintain a calorie deficit for fat loss.

- Muscle preservation: When you're in a calorie deficit for fat loss, there's a risk of losing muscle mass along with fat. Sufficient sleep helps preserve muscle mass by supporting protein synthesis and minimizing muscle breakdown. This is essential for maintaining a muscular physique during the fat-loss process.

- Recovery and workout performance: Quality sleep enhances recovery from workouts, allowing you to perform at your best during exercise sessions. Improved performance leads to greater calorie expenditure and the potential for more intense fat-burning workouts.

- Stress reduction: Lack of sleep can increase stress levels and trigger the release of cortisol, a hormone associated with fat storage, particularly in the abdominal region. Managing stress through adequate sleep can help control cortisol levels and support healthy fat loss.

Individual sleep needs can vary, but most adults require 7-9 hours of quality sleep each night. Prioritizing sufficient and restful sleep supports your muscle-building efforts and promotes successful fat loss by optimizing hormonal balance, muscle recovery, energy levels, and overall well-being.

Strategies for Improving Sleep Quality

Adequate sleep is crucial for optimal health, muscle building, and fat loss. It's during sleep that our bodies recover, repair tissues, and consolidate memories. Unfortunately, many people struggle with sleep-related issues that can negatively impact their well-being and fitness goals. To improve sleep quality, consider implementing the following strategies:

1. Establish a consistent sleep schedule: Set a regular sleep schedule by going to bed and waking up at the same time every day, including weekends. This helps regulate your body's internal clock and promotes a more consistent sleep-wake cycle.

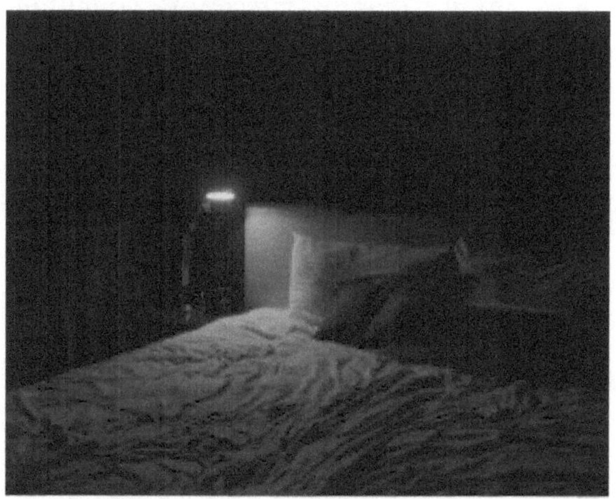

2. Create a sleep-friendly environment: Make your sleep environment conducive to rest by ensuring it is dark, quiet, and cool. Consider using blackout curtains, earplugs, or a white noise machine to block out any disruptive elements that may interfere with your sleep.

3. Develop a relaxing bedtime routine: Establish a relaxing routine leading up to bedtime to signal to your body that it's time to unwind. This can include activities like reading a book, taking a warm bath, practicing gentle stretching or yoga, or mindfulness practices and meditation.

4. Limit exposure to electronic devices: Minimize exposure to electronic devices, such as smartphones, tablets, or laptops, at least one hour before bed. The blue light emitted by these devices can disrupt your sleep-wake cycle by suppressing the production of melatonin, a hormone that regulates sleep.

5. Create a sleep-friendly bedroom: Ensure your bedroom is primarily associated with sleep and relaxation. Avoid using your bed for activities like work or watching TV, as this can confuse your brain and make it harder to wind down. Reserve your bed for sleep and intimate activities only.

6. Manage stress levels: High levels of stress can make it difficult to fall asleep and stay asleep. Incorporate stress management techniques into your daily routine, such as meditation, deep breathing exercises, journaling, or engaging in calming hobbies, to help relax your mind and body before bed. Also, avoid being on platforms that trigger you emotionally. It doesn't serve you in any way and is just stupid.

7. Limit caffeine and stimulants: Avoid consuming caffeinated beverages or stimulants close to bedtime, as they can interfere with your ability to fall asleep. Opt for decaffeinated options or herbal teas instead.

8. Exercise regularly: Regular exercise can promote better sleep, but try to complete your workout earlier in the day. Intense exercise close to bedtime may increase alertness and make it harder to fall asleep. Aim to finish your workouts at least a few hours before bed.

9. Create a comfortable sleep environment: Invest in a supportive mattress, pillows, and bedding that promote comfort and good sleep posture. Experiment with different sleep positions to find the one that works best for you.

10. Avoid heavy meals and alcohol before bed: Eating heavy meals or consuming alcohol close to bedtime can disrupt sleep patterns and lead to discomfort. Opt for lighter, easily digestible meals in the evening and avoid excessive alcohol consumption.

11. Consider relaxation techniques: Explore relaxation techniques like progressive muscle relaxation, guided imagery, mindfulness practice, or aromatherapy to calm your mind and relax your body before bed. These techniques can help reduce anxiety and promote more restful sleep.

Improving sleep quality is a gradual process, and it may take time to establish new habits and routines. Experiment with different strategies and find what works best for you. By prioritizing quality sleep, you'll enhance your recovery, support your fitness goals, and improve your overall wellness.

Active Recovery & Its Benefits

Active recovery is a strategy used to facilitate the recovery process after intense exercise or physical activity. Unlike complete rest, active recovery involves engaging in low-intensity exercises or activities that promote blood flow, muscle relaxation, and overall physical and mental restoration. Active recovery can have several benefits for athletes and fitness enthusiasts:

1. Enhanced muscle recovery: Engaging in light exercises, such as gentle stretching, walking, or low-impact activities, stimulates blood flow to the muscles. This increased circulation helps deliver oxygen and nutrients to the muscles, removing metabolic waste products and promoting faster recovery.

2. Reduction of muscle soreness: Active recovery can help alleviate muscle soreness and stiffness commonly experienced after intense exercise. The gentle movements and increased blood flow help flush out lactic acid and other byproducts, reducing inflammation and promoting muscle repair.

3. Maintenance of range of motion and flexibility: Incorporating active recovery exercises that focus on mobility and flexibility helps maintain joint range of motion and prevents muscle tightness. Activities like yoga, Pilates, or gentle stretching routines can help improve flexibility and keep the body supple.

4. Injury prevention: Active recovery sessions can help reduce the risk of injuries by addressing muscle imbalances and promoting proper movement patterns.

5. Mental rejuvenation: Active recovery not only benefits the body but also provides an opportunity for mental rejuvenation. Engaging in light physical activity, such as going for a walk in nature or

practicing mindfulness exercises, can help reduce stress, promote relaxation, and improve mood and mental well-being.

6. Active recovery as a training stimulus: Incorporating active recovery sessions into your training program can serve as a valuable training stimulus. By engaging in low-intensity exercises, you stimulate muscle fibers without overtaxing them, promoting active regeneration and improving overall fitness levels.

7. Improved workout performance: Active recovery can enhance subsequent workout performance by promoting better circulation, reducing muscle fatigue, and enhancing recovery between training sessions. By incorporating active recovery into your routine, you can maintain a higher level of overall performance and avoid burnout.

8. Long-term sustainability: Active recovery plays a vital role in promoting long-term sustainability in training programs. By allowing the body to recover and recharge, it helps prevent overtraining and reduces the risk of chronic fatigue or injury, allowing for consistent progress and sustainable training practices.

Here are some examples of active recovery exercises and activities:

1. Light jogging or brisk walking: Going for a gentle jog or brisk walk can help increase blood flow, elevate heart rate slightly, and promote active recovery without excessive stress on the muscles.

2. Cycling: Taking a leisurely bike ride or using a stationary bike at a low resistance level can be an effective way to engage in active recovery while minimizing the impact on the joints.

3. Swimming: Swimming or water-based exercises provide a low-impact, full-body workout that promotes muscle relaxation, cardiovascular health, and overall recovery.

4. Yoga or Pilates: Engaging in yoga or Pilates sessions focuses on gentle stretching, improving flexibility, and promoting relaxation. These activities can help alleviate muscle tightness and enhance overall body mobility.

5. Light resistance training: Incorporating light resistance exercises with minimal weights or resistance bands can help maintain muscle activation and stimulate blood flow without causing excessive muscle damage or fatigue.

6. Foam rolling or self-myofascial release: Using a foam roller or other self-massage tools can help release muscle tension and knots, promoting muscle recovery and relaxation.

7. Stretching and mobility exercises: Performing static stretches or dynamic mobility exercises for major muscle groups can improve flexibility, range of motion, and relieve muscle tightness.

8. Low-impact group classes: Participating in low-impact group fitness classes, such as gentle aerobics, dance-based workouts, or tai chi, can provide a fun and social way to engage in active recovery.

9. Hiking or nature walks: Taking a leisurely hike or nature walk allows you to engage in light physical activity while enjoying the outdoors and benefiting from the calming effects of nature.

10. Mindfulness activities: Engaging in mindfulness practices, such as meditation, deep breathing exercises, or gentle yoga flows, can promote mental relaxation, reduce stress, and support overall well-being during the recovery process.

Remember, the key is to keep the intensity low and focus on promoting relaxation, blood flow, and overall recovery. Choose activities that you enjoy and that align with your preferences and fitness level. By incorporating active recovery into your routine, you'll optimize your recovery, support your training progress, and enhance your overall fitness journey.

When incorporating active recovery into your routine, remember to listen to your body and adjust the intensity and duration of the activities based on your current fitness level and recovery needs. Active recovery should be gentle and enjoyable, providing a break from high-intensity workouts while still promoting physical and mental well-being.

Active recovery is a valuable component of any training program. It offers numerous benefits, including improved muscle recovery, reduced muscle soreness, injury prevention, mental rejuvenation, and enhanced workout performance. By prioritizing active recovery, you'll optimize your training outcomes, support long-term progress, and maintain a healthy and balanced approach to fitness.

Sleep & Recovery Hacks

In this section, we will look at different ways to optimize sleep beyond the basics, how to recover from lost sleep, and other tips and hacks to recover to our fullest potential.

The circadian rhythm and how to optimize it:

The circadian rhythm is a natural internal clock that regulates various physiological processes in our bodies, including sleep-wake cycles, hormone production, metabolism, and cognitive functions. It follows a 24-hour cycle, responding primarily to light and darkness cues from the environment. However, it also responds to things such as exercise, temperature, stimulation and caffeine, stress, and more. Hormones such as cortisol and melatonin are majorly linked to the circadian rhythm. Melatonin makes you feel sleepy and relaxed, while cortisol makes you more alert and wakeful.

Optimizing our circadian rhythm can have profound effects on our overall health, wellness, and performance. Here are some strategies to help you optimize your circadian rhythm:

1. Maintain a consistent sleep schedule: Try to go to bed and wake up at the same time every day, including weekends. This regular sleep pattern helps align your body's internal clock, making it easier to fall asleep and wake up naturally.

2. Expose yourself to natural light: Get exposure to natural sunlight during the day, especially in the morning. Natural light helps regulate your circadian rhythm by signaling to your body that it's daytime, promoting alertness and wakefulness. Spend time outdoors or open curtains and blinds to let sunlight into your living and working spaces.

3. Minimize exposure to artificial light at night: Limit your exposure to bright screens, such as smartphones, tablets, and computers, especially before bedtime. The blue light emitted by these devices can suppress the production of melatonin, a hormone that regulates sleep. Consider using blue light filters or wearing blue light-blocking glasses in the evening to reduce the impact of artificial light on your circadian rhythm.

4. Create a sleep-friendly environment: Make your bedroom conducive to quality sleep. Keep the room cool, dark, and quiet. Use curtains or blinds to block out external light, and consider using earplugs or a white noise machine to minimize disruptive noises. A comfortable mattress, pillows, and bedding can also contribute to better sleep quality.

5. Establish a relaxing bedtime routine: Develop a consistent wind-down routine before bed to signal to your body that it's time to sleep. Engage in activities that promote relaxation, such as reading a book, taking a warm bath, practicing gentle stretching or yoga, or listening to soothing music. Avoid stimulating activities or stressful situations close to bedtime.

6. Be mindful of caffeine and stimulant intake: Limit your consumption of caffeine, especially in the afternoon and evening. Caffeine can interfere with your sleep quality and disrupt your circadian rhythm. Be aware of other stimulants, such as nicotine and certain medications, which can also affect your sleep. Also, if possible, you shouldn't consume any caffeine or other stimulants too early in the day. Wait for at least 60-90 minutes after waking up.

7. Regular exercise: Engaging in regular physical activity, preferably earlier in the day, can help regulate your circadian rhythm. Exercise promotes alertness during the day and can contribute to better sleep

quality at night. However, avoid intense workouts close to bedtime, as they may interfere with your ability to fall asleep.

8. Consider chronotherapy: In certain cases, such as when adjusting to a new time zone or dealing with circadian rhythm disorders, chronotherapy may be beneficial. This involves gradually shifting your sleep-wake schedule over several days to align with the desired time zone or to reset your internal clock.

By optimizing your circadian rhythm, you can enhance your sleep quality, increase daytime alertness, improve mood and cognitive function, and support overall health and well-being. Experiment with these strategies and find the ones that work best for you in establishing healthy sleep habits and maintaining a synchronized circadian rhythm.

Relaxing Drinks, Teas, and Tricks for a Restful Night's Sleep

1. Chamomile Tea: Chamomile tea is well-known for its calming properties. It contains compounds that promote relaxation and can help reduce anxiety. Enjoying a cup of chamomile tea before bed can be a soothing ritual that signals to your body it's time to wind down and prepare for sleep.

2. Warm Milk: Warm milk has been a popular bedtime beverage for ages. It contains an amino acid called tryptophan, which is a precursor to serotonin, a neurotransmitter that promotes relaxation and sleep. Heating the milk enhances its soothing effect, making it a comforting and calming drink before bed.

3. Herbal Teas: Besides chamomile, several other herbal teas can aid in relaxation and sleep. Lavender tea has gentle sedative properties and can help calm the mind and promote sleepiness. Peppermint tea and lemon balm tea are also known for their relaxing effects.

4. Valerian Root Tea: Valerian root has long been used as a natural remedy for insomnia and sleep disturbances. It can help improve sleep quality and reduce the time it takes to fall asleep. Valerian root tea, which is made from the dried roots of the valerian plant, can be a beneficial addition to your nighttime routine.

5. Magnesium-Rich Drinks: Magnesium is an essential mineral that plays a role in promoting relaxation and quality sleep. Consuming drinks rich in magnesium, such as magnesium-fortified water, herbal magnesium supplements, or natural sources like magnesium-rich mineral water, can help relax your muscles and calm your nervous system.

6. Tart Cherry Juice: Tart cherry juice is a natural source of melatonin, a hormone that regulates sleep-wake cycles. Drinking a small glass of tart cherry juice in the evening may help increase melatonin levels, promoting better sleep.

7. Decaffeinated Herbal Infusions: Herbal infusions that are free of caffeine, such as lemon verbena, passionflower, or valerian root infusions, can provide a soothing and relaxing experience without the stimulating effects of caffeine.

8. Relaxation Techniques: Besides beverages, incorporating relaxation techniques into your evening routine can help prepare your body and mind for sleep. Consider practicing deep breathing exercises, mindfulness meditation, gentle stretching, or progressive muscle relaxation. These techniques can promote relaxation, reduce stress, and enhance your ability to fall and stay asleep.

9. Sleeping with socks: Sleeping with socks on might sound weird, but it has been shown to improve circulation and make your body cooler, which helps you have a more restful night.

10. Blackout curtains: If your room is too bright, you won't have a deep sleep and you'll probably have trouble falling asleep too. You can either use blackout curtains to block out the light from outside or achieve the same result with a sleeping mask.

Everyone responds differently to various drinks and relaxation techniques, so it's important to experiment and find what works best for you. It's also a good idea to consult with a healthcare professional if you have any specific concerns or if you are taking medications that may interact with certain drinks or herbs. Ultimately, creating a peaceful and relaxing bedtime routine that includes your preferred drinks and relaxation techniques can significantly contribute to better sleep and overall health.

Boosting Energy and Alertness: Drinks and Strategies for Daytime Vitality

In our fast-paced world, maintaining high energy levels and staying alert throughout the day is crucial for productivity and overall well-being. While a good night's sleep and healthy lifestyle habits are fundamental, some additional strategies and drinks can help boost energy and enhance alertness. This chapter explores various approaches to support daytime vitality, including beverages and practical techniques that promote sustained energy levels and mental focus.

1. Hydration for Energy:

One of the simplest and often overlooked factors in maintaining energy levels is proper hydration. Dehydration can lead to fatigue and decreased cognitive function. Make it a habit to drink an adequate amount of water throughout the day, aiming for at least 8-10 glasses. You can also include hydrating beverages like herbal teas, infused water, and coconut water to replenish electrolytes and provide a refreshing boost.

2. Energizing Drinks:

a) Green Tea: Known for its moderate caffeine content and abundant antioxidants, green tea provides a gentle energy lift without the jitters associated with coffee. It enhances mental alertness and has been linked to improved cognitive function and fat metabolism.

b) Matcha: This powdered form of green tea offers a concentrated dose of antioxidants and a unique combination of caffeine and L-theanine. Matcha promotes sustained energy and mental clarity while inducing a calming effect.

c) Coffee: The primary ingredient in coffee that provides its stimulating effects is caffeine. When consumed, caffeine quickly enters the bloodstream and travels to the brain, where it interacts with receptors that regulate the sleep-wake cycle. By blocking the action of adenosine, a neurotransmitter that promotes relaxation and drowsiness, caffeine helps to keep us alert and awake.

3. Balanced Nutrition:

Fueling your body with a well-balanced diet is vital for sustained energy levels. Include nutrient-dense foods that provide a steady release of energy throughout the day, such as whole grains, lean proteins, fruits, and vegetables. Avoid excessive consumption of sugary or processed foods, as they can lead to energy crashes and sluggishness.

4. Mindful Movement:

Engaging in regular physical activity can increase alertness and boost energy levels. Incorporate short bursts of exercise or movement breaks throughout the day to stimulate blood flow, oxygenate the brain, and enhance mental focus. Activities like stretching, brisk walking, or even a quick dance session can provide an instant energy boost.

5. Natural Supplements:

Certain natural supplements, when used responsibly and under professional guidance, may support energy and mental clarity. Examples include ginseng, rhodiola rosea, ashwagandha, and B-vitamin complexes. It's essential to consult with a healthcare professional or nutritionist before incorporating supplements into your routine. Focus on getting the basics right, and only add supplements if you have mastered them.

6. Optimizing Light Exposure:

Natural light exposure plays a crucial role in regulating the circadian rhythm, which affects energy levels and alertness. Spend time outdoors during daylight hours, allowing your body to absorb natural sunlight. If natural light is limited, consider using light therapy devices that mimic daylight to help regulate your internal body clock.

Boosting energy and maintaining alertness throughout the day requires a holistic approach. By incorporating the strategies mentioned above and incorporating energy-enhancing drinks into your routine, you can optimize your vitality and improve overall performance. Experiment with different techniques and beverages to find what works best for you, always prioritizing healthy habits and listening to your body's needs.

Remember to consult with healthcare professionals or nutritionists before making any significant changes to your diet or introducing new supplements.

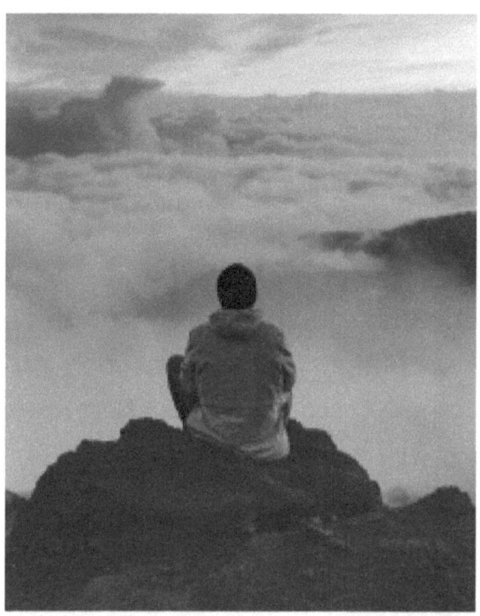

Yoga Nidra: Deep Rest and Recovery for Daytime Sleep Deprivation

In our fast-paced modern lives, it's not uncommon to experience daytime sleep deprivation due to various reasons. When traditional sleep isn't possible, finding alternative methods to recover and restore energy becomes essential. One powerful practice that can help in this regard is Yoga Nidra. Let's explore what Yoga Nidra is and how it can aid in recovering from lost sleep during the day.

Yoga Nidra, also known as yogic sleep, is a guided meditation technique that induces a state of deep relaxation and promotes physical, mental, and emotional restoration. It is different from traditional sleep as it allows the practitioner to experience a state of conscious awareness while the body remains in a relaxed and restful state. This practice involves systematically moving through different stages of relaxation, sensory withdrawal, and visualization, leading to a state of profound rest.

Here's how Yoga Nidra can help recover from lost sleep during the day:

1. Deep Relaxation: Yoga Nidra takes you into a state of deep relaxation, allowing your body and mind to release tension and stress. This state of profound rest can help rejuvenate and recharge, providing a similar level of rest as sleep.

2. Stress reduction: Sleep deprivation can elevate stress levels, leading to physical and mental fatigue. Yoga Nidra promotes relaxation and activates the body's relaxation response, reducing stress hormones and promoting a sense of calm and well-being.

3. Enhanced focus and clarity: Daytime sleep deprivation can impair cognitive function, making it difficult to concentrate and stay focused. Yoga Nidra helps clear mental clutter and enhances mental clarity, allowing you to regain focus and improve productivity.

4. Rebalancing energy levels: Yoga Nidra works with the body's subtle energy system, helping to balance and restore energy levels. It can help alleviate feelings of sluggishness, lethargy, and low motivation that often accompany sleep deprivation.

5. Improved mood and emotional well-being: Lack of sleep can negatively impact mood, leading to irritability, mood swings, and increased emotional reactivity. Yoga Nidra promotes a sense of calmness, stability, and emotional balance, helping to improve overall emotional well-being.

6. Restoring mind-body connection: Sleep deprivation can disrupt the harmony between the mind and body. Yoga Nidra facilitates a

deep connection between body, mind, and breath, promoting a sense of unity and inner balance.

7. Enhancing self-awareness and introspection: The practice of Yoga Nidra encourages self-reflection and introspection. It allows you to explore your thoughts, emotions, and experiences, leading to a deeper understanding of yourself and promoting personal growth.

To incorporate Yoga Nidra into your day for sleep recovery:

1. Find a quiet and comfortable space where you can lie down or sit in a relaxed position.

2. Use guided audio recordings or attend a Yoga Nidra class to be led through the practice.

3. Follow the instructions given, which typically involve progressive relaxation, breath awareness, visualization, and conscious intention setting.

4. Allow yourself to fully surrender to the practice, letting go of tension, thoughts, and worries.

5. Practice regularly, even for short durations, to experience the cumulative benefits over time.

Remember, while Yoga Nidra can provide restorative effects and help recover from lost sleep during the day, it should not replace the importance of regular, quality sleep. It can be a valuable tool to supplement your sleep routine and provide rejuvenation when traditional sleep is limited. Prioritize a balanced sleep schedule and healthy sleep habits for optimal well-being and vitality.

Non-sleep Deep Rest (NSDR): Rejuvenating the Mind and Body without Sleep

In our busy lives, finding time for proper sleep can sometimes be challenging. However, there are alternative practices that can provide deep rest and rejuvenation, even when traditional sleep is limited. One such approach is Non-Sleep Deep Rest (NSDR). Let's explore what NSDR is and how it can help you replenish and recharge.

NSDR refers to intentional practices that induce a state of deep restfulness and relaxation without actually sleeping. These practices aim to provide the mind and body with an opportunity to recover, regenerate, and revitalize, promoting overall well-being. Here are some NSDR techniques and practices that can help you experience deep rest:

1. Meditation: Meditation is a powerful practice for achieving deep rest and relaxation. By focusing your attention and calming the mind, meditation can induce a state of profound tranquility, reducing mental chatter and promoting mental clarity and inner calmness.

2. Breathwork: Various breathwork techniques, such as deep diaphragmatic breathing or alternate nostril breathing, can activate the body's relaxation response and help release tension and stress. Conscious breathing can be practiced anywhere, providing a quick and effective way to achieve a state of deep rest.

3. Progressive Muscle Relaxation (PMR): PMR involves systematically tensing and relaxing different muscle groups, promoting physical relaxation and releasing muscle tension. This technique allows you to consciously relax the body and achieve a state of deep restfulness.

4. Yoga Nidra: As mentioned earlier, Yoga Nidra is a guided practice that induces a state of deep relaxation. It combines elements of breath awareness, body scanning, and visualization to promote physical, mental, and emotional restoration.

5. Mindfulness: Practicing mindfulness involves being fully present in the current moment, observing thoughts, sensations, and emotions without judgment. By cultivating a state of mindfulness, you can experience a sense of deep rest and calmness.

6. Sensory Deprivation: Creating an environment free from external stimuli can help facilitate deep rest. Techniques such as floating in a sensory deprivation tank or using an eye mask, earplugs, or a quiet and dimly lit space can help minimize sensory input and promote relaxation.

7. Sound Therapy: Listening to calming and soothing sounds, such as nature sounds, instrumental music, or white noise, can induce a state of relaxation and provide a sense of deep restfulness.

8. Visualization and Imagery: Engaging in guided visualization exercises, where you imagine serene and peaceful scenes, can help relax the mind and evoke a state of deep rest and tranquility.

To incorporate NSDR practices into your routine:

1. Set aside dedicated time for deep rest and relaxation each day, even if it's just a few minutes.

2. Choose the NSDR technique that resonates with you the most and aligns with your preferences and needs.

3. Create a quiet, comfortable, and distraction-free environment to enhance the deep rest experience.

4. Consistency is key. Regular practice will help you reap the benefits of NSDR over time.

While NSDR practices can provide rejuvenation and replenishment, they should not replace the importance of regular, quality sleep. They can be complementary tools to support you, especially during periods when sleep is limited. Prioritize a balanced sleep schedule and healthy sleep habits alongside NSDR practices for optimal physical, mental, and emotional vitality.

The Ultradian Cycle: Optimizing Sleep for Enhanced Rest and Productivity

Our sleep patterns are influenced by various biological rhythms, one of which is the ultradian cycle. Understanding this cycle can help us optimize our sleep and enhance our overall rest and productivity. Let's delve into what the ultradian cycle is and how we can make the most of it.

The ultradian cycle refers to a recurring pattern of physiological and brain activity that occurs in cycles of approximately 90 to 120 minutes throughout the day and night. These cycles consist of alternating periods of high-frequency brain activity (when we are awake and alert) and low-frequency brain activity (when we are in a state of rest and relaxation). By aligning our sleep with the ultradian cycle, we can tap into our natural rhythms and experience more restorative sleep.

Here are some strategies to optimize your sleep based on the ultradian cycle:

1. Honor Your Sleep Cycles: Aim to get a sufficient amount of sleep by allowing yourself to complete multiple sleep cycles. Each cycle

typically lasts around 90 minutes, so targeting 7-9 hours of sleep will allow you to go through several complete cycles and wake up at the end of a cycle, feeling more refreshed.

2. Plan Your Wake-Up Time: Rather than focusing solely on your bedtime, consider the time you need to wake up and work backward to determine your optimal bedtime. This approach ensures you complete full sleep cycles and wake up during a phase of lighter sleep, making it easier to transition into wakefulness.

3. Nap Wisely: Leverage the power of napping to recharge and boost productivity. Since the ultradian cycle repeats throughout the day, taking short power naps of 20-30 minutes can help you tap into periods of low-frequency brain activity and emerge feeling revitalized. My recommendation on when to nap is right around noon (lunchtime) and avoid taking naps after 2 pm as it may affect your ability to fall asleep at a reasonable time later that night.

4. Listen to Your Body's Signals: Pay attention to your natural energy fluctuations throughout the day. Notice when you feel a dip in alertness or focus and take advantage of these moments to rest or engage in a short relaxation practice. By aligning your activities with your body's ultradian rhythm, you can optimize your energy and productivity.

5. Create Sleep-Friendly Environments: Design your bedroom and sleep environment to promote restful sleep. Keep the room cool, dark, and quiet, and minimize distractions that could disrupt your sleep cycles. Consider using white noise machines or earplugs to create a soothing atmosphere.

6. Practice Sleep Hygiene: Adopt healthy sleep habits to support your body's natural sleep-wake cycle. Establish a consistent sleep schedule, avoid stimulants like caffeine close to bedtime, limit

exposure to screens and electronic devices, and engage in relaxing pre-sleep routines to prepare your mind and body for rest.

7. Experiment and Adjust: Recognize that individual sleep needs can vary. Pay attention to how you feel upon waking and throughout the day, and adjust your sleep patterns accordingly. Experiment with different sleep durations and wake-up times to find what works best for you.

By aligning our sleep patterns with the natural rhythms of the ultradian cycle, we can optimize our rest and enhance our daytime performance.

The Importance of Rest Days in Your Training Program

Rest days are often overlooked or undervalued in fitness programs, but they play a crucial role in achieving optimal results and maintaining long-term progress. Whether you're engaging in intense weightlifting, endurance training, or any other form of physical activity, incorporating regular rest days into your training program is essential for your overall health, recovery, and performance. Let's explore why rest days are so important:

Recovery and Repair: Rest days allow your body to recover and repair from the stress and micro-tears caused by exercise. During workouts, your muscles undergo a breakdown process, and it's during rest that they rebuild and become stronger. Adequate rest gives your body the time it needs to repair damaged tissues, replenish energy stores, and restore balance.

Injury Prevention: Overtraining and lack of rest can increase the risk of injuries. Without proper recovery, your muscles, tendons, and joints become fatigued and more susceptible to strains, sprains, and other injuries. Rest days provide an opportunity for your body to heal, reduce inflammation, and prevent injuries.

Muscular and Strength Development: Rest days are essential for muscle growth and strength development. While exercise stimulates muscle growth, it's during rest that your muscles grow in size and strength. Rest days allow your muscles to adapt to the stress of training, leading to improved muscle fiber recruitment and enhanced performance.

Mental and Emotional Well-being: Physical activity places stress on both your body and mind. Rest days provide a mental break from the demands of training, allowing you to recharge mentally and emotionally. Taking time off from structured workouts can help reduce mental fatigue, prevent burnout, and enhance your overall well-being.

Hormonal Balance: Intense exercise can disrupt hormonal balance in the body. Rest days help restore hormonal equilibrium, particularly cortisol and testosterone levels. Cortisol, the stress hormone, decreases during rest, while testosterone, an anabolic hormone crucial for muscle growth, increases. This hormonal balance supports muscle recovery, growth, and overall fitness.

Performance Improvement: Adequate rest is essential for maximizing performance gains. Rest days allow your body to adapt and respond to the stress of training, leading to improved strength, endurance, and athletic performance. By incorporating strategic rest days into your program, you allow your body to perform at its best when it matters most.

Long-Term Sustainability: Rest days are crucial for long-term sustainability and preventing burnout. Pushing your body to its limits without adequate recovery can lead to diminished performance, chronic fatigue, and decreased motivation to continue training. Rest days promote a healthy and sustainable approach to fitness, allowing you to enjoy consistent progress over time.

Remember, rest days don't mean you have to be completely sedentary. Active recovery, such as light stretching, yoga, or low-intensity activities, can still be beneficial on rest days. Listen to your body, pay attention to signs of fatigue or overtraining, and adjust your training schedule accordingly.

Incorporating rest days into your training program is a key component of achieving optimal fitness results, preventing injuries, and maintaining long-term progress.

How to Manage Stress For Better Recovery and Rest

In our fast-paced and demanding world, stress has become a common companion in our daily lives. The constant pressures and responsibilities can take a toll on our physical and mental well-being, affecting our ability to recover and rest effectively. Therefore, it's essential to develop strategies to manage stress and promote better recovery and rest. Here are some key approaches to help you manage stress effectively:

Realize That Every Great Person Went Through Stress, You Need to Learn How to Go Through Hard Things: Realize that the person you aspire to be like has become the person he or she is by doing hard and stressful things. Instead of focusing so much on stress, which in turn makes you stress even more, focus more on achieving your goals and improving your performance and life. When you are so focused on something else, stress becomes less noticeable to you.

Self-Care: Make self-care a habit in your daily routine. Engage in activities that bring you joy and help you relax, such as reading, taking a bath, practicing mindfulness or meditation, listening to calming music, or spending time in nature. Self-care allows you to recharge and refocus, enhancing your ability to handle stress.

Practice Stress-Relieving Techniques: Explore different stress-relieving techniques to find what works best for you. Deep breathing exercises, progressive muscle relaxation, and guided imagery are effective practices for reducing stress and promoting a state of relaxation. Experiment with different techniques and incorporate them into your daily routine.

Regular Exercise: Engaging in regular physical activity is an excellent stress management tool. Exercise releases endorphins, which are known as "feel-good" hormones that help reduce stress and improve mood. Find a form of exercise that you enjoy, whether it's jogging, cycling, dancing, or practicing yoga, and make it a part of your routine.

Time Management: Poor time management can contribute to stress and overwhelm. Take control of your schedule by prioritizing tasks, setting realistic goals, and practicing effective time management techniques. By allocating dedicated time for rest, relaxation, and recovery activities, you can better manage stress and create a balanced lifestyle.

Social Support: Cultivate a strong support system of family, friends, or a community that understands and supports you. Sharing your thoughts, feelings, and concerns with trusted individuals can help alleviate stress. Seek support when needed and foster meaningful connections that provide a sense of belonging and emotional well-being.

Healthy Sleep Habits: Quality sleep is crucial for stress management and overall well-being. Establish a consistent sleep routine and create a sleep-friendly environment. Practice good sleep hygiene by avoiding stimulating activities before bedtime, limiting exposure to electronic devices, and creating a calm and comfortable sleep environment. Prioritizing restful sleep will significantly improve your ability to cope with stress.

Mindfulness and Mind-Body Practices: Incorporate mindfulness and mind-body practices into your daily routine. These practices, such as meditation, yoga, tai chi, and qigong, help cultivate present-moment awareness, reduce stress, and enhance relaxation. By connecting your mind and body, you can promote a state of calm and balance.

Journaling: Journaling is a powerful tool that can help you relieve stress, increase mindfulness, and boost motivation. By putting your thoughts and feelings on paper, you gain clarity and a deeper understanding of yourself. It allows you to process emotions, identify patterns, and find solutions to challenges. Journaling promotes self-reflection, gratitude, and goal-setting, enhancing your overall well-being. It's a simple practice with profound benefits, offering a space for self-expression and personal growth.

Managing stress is an ongoing process that requires self-awareness, practice, and patience. Each person's stress management strategies may vary, so it's important to find what works best for you. By implementing these approaches into your daily life, you can effectively manage stress and promote better recovery and rest.

How Much Sleep Do You Need?

The amount of sleep you need can vary depending on various factors, including age, lifestyle, and individual differences. While there isn't a one-size-fits-all answer, understanding your sleep needs is essential for overall health and well-being.

On average, adults generally require between 7 to 9 hours of sleep per night to function optimally. 7-9 hours of sleep, not 7-9 hours in bed. There's a thing called sleep efficiency, which is how much of the time you are in bed you spend sleeping. A "good" sleep efficiency is 80-85%, which means if you want to sleep 8 hours you should dedicate approximately 9 hours in bed. And that's just assuming your sleep is good and there's nothing psychologically wrong with you.

However, some individuals may need slightly more or less sleep to feel fully rested and refreshed. It's important to listen to your body and pay attention to how you feel after different amounts of sleep.

Factors such as physical activity, stress levels, and overall health can influence your sleep needs. Athletes or individuals engaging in intense physical activity may require additional sleep to support muscle recovery and repair. Likewise, individuals experiencing high levels of stress may benefit from additional sleep to promote emotional and mental well-being.

It's worth noting that quality of sleep is equally important as quantity. Factors like sleep environment, sleep hygiene practices, and sleep disorders can impact the quality of your sleep, even if you spend the recommended time in bed. Prioritizing both the duration and quality of your sleep is key to achieving optimal rest and functioning during the day.

To determine your individual sleep needs, pay attention to how you feel after different amounts of sleep and adjust your sleep schedule accordingly. Experiment with different sleep durations and establish a consistent sleep routine to promote a healthy sleep-wake cycle.

Remember, everyone is unique, and finding the right amount of sleep for you may require some trial and error. If you don't sleep enough for one day, don't worry or start stressing. Stressing about sleep is one of the worst things you can do. Listen to your body, prioritize sleep as an essential part of your self-care routine, and make adjustments to ensure you're getting the restorative sleep you need to thrive.

VI: Common Misconceptions & Myths

Myths and misconceptions have a sneaky way of infiltrating the world of fitness and nutrition, clouding our judgment and hindering our progress. These misguided beliefs often stem from misinformation, popular trends, or even well-intentioned but misinterpreted advice. Unfortunately, these myths can hold us back from reaching our true potential and achieving our goals. It's time to set the record straight and unravel the truth behind these common misconceptions.

Behind the flashy headlines and bold claims, lies the truth obscured by myths. Many individuals fall victim to misconceptions that promise quick fixes, shortcuts, or magical solutions. However, as we navigate through the labyrinth of fitness and nutrition, it becomes apparent that success is built on a foundation of knowledge, consistency, and evidence-based practices.

In this chapter, we will shed light on some of the most prevalent myths and misconceptions that permeate the fitness and nutrition industry. By diving deep into each misconception, we aim to unravel the truth, empowering you to make informed decisions and adopt strategies that will lead to sustainable progress.

Myths and misconceptions can create self-imposed limitations, hindering our ability to make positive changes. By debunking these falsehoods, we hope to liberate you from the shackles of misinformation and open up a world of possibilities. Understanding the truth behind common misconceptions allows you to approach your fitness and nutrition journey with clarity, confidence, and the ability to discern fact from fiction.

By addressing these myths head-on, we aim to arm you with accurate information and dispel the misconceptions that may be holding you back. Armed with the truth, you can navigate the fitness and nutrition landscape with confidence, making choices that align with your goals and promote long-term success.

Spot Reduction

Many people have fallen victim to the myth that performing specific exercises, such as crunches or leg lifts, can target fat loss in specific areas of the body. This misconception suggests that by focusing on certain exercises, individuals can tone and sculpt specific muscles or eliminate fat from specific problem areas. However, it's essential to understand the truth behind this myth and the factors that contribute to overall body fat reduction and muscle toning.

Debunking the Myth of Spot Reduction:

1. Body Fat Distribution: Our bodies store fat in different areas based on genetic predispositions and hormonal influences. Targeting specific exercises for a particular body part does not directly burn fat in that area. Fat loss occurs throughout the body as a result of overall energy expenditure and calorie deficit.

2. Energy Balance and Fat Loss: To lose fat, you need to create an energy deficit by burning more calories than you consume. This deficit encourages the body to tap into its fat stores for energy. While exercises can contribute to overall calorie burn, they do not selectively burn fat from specific regions.

3. Muscle Toning and Overall Body Composition: The idea of toning or shaping a muscle refers to increasing muscle definition and decreasing body fat percentage. To achieve this, it's necessary to build muscle mass through resistance training exercises that target multiple muscle groups. Combining strength training with proper nutrition and cardiovascular exercise helps improve overall body composition and create a leaner appearance.

4. Genetics and Body Composition: Each individual has a unique genetic makeup that determines where they tend to store or lose fat.

Unfortunately, we cannot control the specific areas from which fat is burned. It is important to focus on overall fat loss and building lean muscle mass to improve body composition and achieve a more balanced physique.

Spot reduction is a common myth in the fitness industry. The reality is that targeting specific exercises for certain body parts does not lead to localized fat loss or muscle toning. Instead, the key lies in maintaining a healthy lifestyle that incorporates a well-rounded fitness routine, including resistance training, cardiovascular exercise, and a balanced diet. By focusing on overall fat loss and improving body composition, you can achieve your fitness goals and develop a more balanced and aesthetic physique.

The Truth About Detox Diets

In recent years, detox diets and cleanses have gained significant popularity as a way to cleanse the body of toxins and promote better health. However, it's important to understand that the concept of detoxing through specific diets or cleanses is not supported by scientific evidence.

The premise behind detox diets is that they help remove toxins from the body, thereby improving overall health and well-being. These diets often involve strict fasting, consuming only specific foods or juices, and sometimes the use of herbal supplements or colon cleanses. Proponents claim that these practices can purify the body, enhance digestion, boost energy levels, and even aid in weight loss.

However, it is crucial to recognize that the body has its own highly efficient detoxification system, primarily centered around the liver and kidneys. These organs work tirelessly to filter and eliminate waste products and toxins from the body. Our bodies are naturally equipped to handle these functions without the need for extreme dietary interventions.

Scientific studies have consistently shown that detox diets and cleanses offer little to no additional benefit in terms of removing toxins from the body. The perceived improvements in health or weight loss experienced during a detox diet are typically short-term and primarily attributed to calorie restriction or temporary changes in eating habits.

Moreover, some detox diets can be extreme and may lack essential nutrients, leading to potential nutritional deficiencies. They can also disrupt the body's natural balance and metabolism, causing negative side effects such as fatigue, dizziness, and digestive issues.

Instead of relying on detox diets, it is far more beneficial to adopt a balanced and sustainable approach to nutrition. Focus on consuming a varied diet rich in whole foods, including fruits, vegetables, lean proteins, whole grains, and healthy fats. This approach provides the body with the necessary nutrients and antioxidants to support its natural detoxification processes.

Remember, our bodies are incredibly resilient and efficient in removing toxins. Rather than subjecting ourselves to restrictive and potentially harmful detox diets, we can promote better health by maintaining a well-rounded and nourishing diet, staying hydrated, getting regular exercise, and prioritizing quality sleep.

Carbohydrates Are Bad

Carbohydrates have long been the subject of much debate and confusion when it comes to nutrition. One common misconception is that all carbohydrates are bad for you and should be avoided. However, it's important to understand that not all carbs are created equal, and demonizing all carbohydrates can lead to an unbalanced and potentially unhealthy diet.

Carbohydrates are one of the three macronutrients essential for our bodies, along with proteins and fats. They provide a primary source of energy and play a vital role in fueling our brain, muscles, and various bodily functions. It's the quality and type of carbohydrates that make the difference in their impact on our health.

Complex carbohydrates, also known as "good carbs," are found in foods like whole grains, legumes, fruits, and vegetables. These carbohydrates contain fiber, vitamins, minerals, and other beneficial compounds that are important for overall health. Complex carbs are digested more slowly, providing a steady release of energy and promoting feelings of fullness and satiety.

On the other hand, simple carbohydrates, often referred to as "bad carbs," are found in sugary beverages, candies, processed snacks, and refined grains. These carbohydrates are quickly digested, leading to rapid spikes in blood sugar levels. Consuming an excess of simple carbs can contribute to weight gain, energy crashes, lower testosterone, and an increased risk of chronic diseases such as type 2 diabetes and heart disease.

By demonizing all carbohydrates, we risk neglecting the essential nutrients and health benefits that complex carbs provide. They are an important part of a balanced diet, offering valuable dietary fiber, vitamins, and minerals that promote digestive health, regulate blood sugar levels, and support overall well-being.

Including complex carbohydrates in our meals can provide sustained energy, improve digestion, and contribute to long-term health. Opt for whole grain products like whole wheat bread, brown rice, quinoa, and oats. Incorporate a variety of colorful fruits and vegetables, which are not only rich in complex carbs but also provide antioxidants and phytochemicals that protect against chronic diseases.

Individual carbohydrate needs may vary depending on factors such as age, activity level, and overall health goals. Consulting with a registered dietitian or nutritionist can help determine the appropriate carbohydrate intake for your specific needs.

Remember, the key is to focus on the quality of carbohydrates we consume rather than demonizing all carbs. By choosing nutrient-dense complex carbs and balancing our overall macronutrient intake, we can enjoy the benefits of carbohydrates while supporting our health and fitness

More Protein = More Muscle

In the pursuit of building muscle and achieving optimal health, many individuals believe that consuming copious amounts of protein is the key to success. However, this popular notion often stems from misconceptions about protein requirements and its role in muscle growth. Let's delve into the truth behind high-protein diets and debunk the myth of excessive protein intake.

1. The Myth: More Protein Means More Muscle:

- Many people believe that consuming excessive protein will automatically lead to increased muscle mass. However, the reality is that muscle growth is a complex process influenced by multiple factors, including overall calorie intake, training stimulus, and protein quality.

- While protein is indeed crucial for muscle repair and growth, exceeding the recommended intake does not guarantee bigger muscles. Consuming excessive protein beyond the body's needs does not provide additional benefits and may even strain the kidneys and liver.

2. The Truth: Optimal Protein Intake:

- The body requires an adequate amount of protein to support muscle growth, repair tissues, and perform vital functions. However, the optimal protein intake depends on various factors such as age, weight, activity level, and overall goals.

- According to reputable health organizations, a general guideline for protein intake for muscle building is around 0.8-1 grams per pound of body weight per day. This amount is sufficient for most healthy individuals to meet their protein needs.

3. Balancing Macronutrients:

- While protein is important, it is crucial to maintain a balanced diet that includes carbohydrates and healthy fats. Carbohydrates provide energy for workouts and overall performance, while fats support hormone production and absorption of fat-soluble vitamins.

- Neglecting carbohydrates and fats in favor of excessive protein can lead to nutrient deficiencies and imbalances, which can adversely affect overall health and hinder performance.

Dispelling the myth of excessive protein intake is vital for understanding the importance of balanced nutrition. While protein is essential for muscle growth and repair, there is no need to overconsume it.

Remember, balance and moderation are key in nutrition.

Cardio Vs. Weightlifting

When it comes to weight loss, many individuals believe that cardio exercises are the only effective way to shed those extra pounds. However, this common misconception overlooks the incredible benefits of incorporating resistance training into your fitness routine. Let's debunk the notion that cardio is the sole path to weight loss and explore the advantages of resistance training for overall fitness and body composition.

Body:

1. The Myth: Cardio Reigns Supreme for Weight Loss:

- It's a prevailing belief that cardio exercises, such as running or cycling, are the primary means of burning calories and losing weight. While cardio certainly plays a role in calorie expenditure, relying solely on cardio may limit your weight loss potential and overlook other important aspects of fitness. For weight loss, you need to be in a caloric deficit. Cardio can help you with that, but your primary focus should be on your nutrition. Trying to out-work a bad diet is unsustainable and much more difficult than just following a good nutrition plan.

2. The Truth: The Power of Resistance Training:

- Resistance training, often associated with lifting weights or using resistance bands, is a game-changer for weight loss and body composition. Building lean muscle mass through resistance training offers several advantages:

- Increased Metabolic Rate: Muscle is metabolically active tissue, meaning it burns more calories at rest than fat. By increasing your muscle mass, you can elevate your resting metabolic rate and burn more calories throughout the day.

- Fat Loss and Body Recomposition: Resistance training helps preserve and build muscle while losing fat, leading to improved body composition. This means you can achieve a leaner, more toned appearance even without substantial weight loss.

- Improved Strength and Function: Resistance training enhances functional strength, making everyday tasks easier and reducing the risk of injuries. It also promotes better bone density and joint health.

- Enhanced Metabolic Adaptations: Unlike cardio, resistance training stimulates the development of lean muscle mass, which has a positive impact on insulin sensitivity, glucose metabolism, and fat utilization.

3. The Synergy of Cardio and Resistance Training:

- While resistance training offers numerous benefits, it's important to note that combining it with cardiovascular exercises creates a well-rounded fitness program.

- Cardiovascular activities elevate heart rate, improve cardiovascular health, and enhance endurance. They also contribute to overall calorie expenditure, making them a valuable addition to a weight loss plan.

- By incorporating both cardio and resistance training, you can optimize fat loss, improve cardiovascular fitness, build strength, and achieve a balanced approach to overall fitness.

Incorporating resistance exercises into your routine alongside cardiovascular activities creates a synergistic effect, allowing you to maximize your weight loss potential, sculpt your body, and improve your health.

Eating After 6 PM

The belief that eating after 6 PM leads to weight gain is a common misconception that has perpetuated dieting culture for years. Many individuals are under the impression that consuming food in the evening automatically translates to extra pounds on the scale. However, it's time to challenge this myth and shed light on the crucial factors that truly impact weight management—overall calorie intake and macronutrient balance.

1. The Myth: Late-Night Eating Causes Weight Gain:

- The belief that eating after 6 PM or late at night leads to weight gain is based on the assumption that our metabolism slows down during the evening hours. However, the body's metabolism remains active and continues to burn calories regardless of the time of day.

- Weight gain occurs when there is a persistent calorie surplus, meaning you consume more calories than your body needs for energy. It is the total calorie intake over time that influences weight gain, not the specific time of the day you consume your meals.

2. The Truth: Calorie Balance and Macronutrient Composition:

- Weight management is primarily determined by the balance between calorie intake and expenditure. To maintain or lose weight, it's essential to focus on creating a calorie deficit—consuming fewer calories than your body needs.

- While the timing of meals is less critical, paying attention to the overall macronutrient balance is vital. Ensuring an adequate intake of proteins, fats, and carbohydrates can help regulate hunger, promote satiety, and support energy levels throughout the day.

3. Factors That Influence Weight Gain:

- Calorie Intake: Whether you eat early or late in the day, consuming an excess of calories over an extended period will lead to weight gain. It's crucial to be mindful of portion sizes and maintain an overall calorie balance that aligns with your goals.

- Food Choices: The types of foods you consume play a significant role in weight management. Highly processed, calorie-dense foods can contribute to weight gain, regardless of the time of day.

- Eating Patterns: Personal eating habits, such as mindless snacking or emotional eating, can impact overall calorie intake. Focusing on mindful eating, listening to hunger and fullness cues, and practicing portion control is essential for weight management.

Instead of fixating on the time of day, prioritize overall calorie intake, food choices, and mindful eating habits. By adopting a well-balanced and sustainable approach to nutrition, you can achieve your weight management goals while enjoying meals at a time that suits your lifestyle. Consult with a fitness professional or registered dietitian for personalized guidance on nutrition and weight management.

Muscle Turning Into Fat

One of the prevailing misconceptions in the fitness world is the belief that muscle can magically transform into fat when you cease exercising. This misconception often discourages individuals from taking breaks or discontinuing their fitness routine. However, it's crucial to understand that muscle and fat are two distinct tissues with different structures and functions. Let's unravel the truth behind this myth and shed light on the realities of muscle and fat.

1. The Myth: Muscle Turns into Fat When You Stop Exercising:

- The notion that muscle turns into fat is a misunderstanding rooted in the changes that occur when exercise habits are altered. When you stop exercising, muscle tissue may decrease in size or undergo atrophy due to reduced stimulus, leading to a loss of muscle mass. Simultaneously, if your calorie intake remains the same, fat may accumulate, increasing body fat percentage.

- However, it's important to note that muscle does not literally transform into fat. They are distinct tissues with different cellular compositions and functions.

2. The Truth: Muscle and Fat Are Different Tissues:

- Muscle Tissue: Muscles are composed of specialized cells called muscle fibers that contract and enable movement. Resistance training and exercise stimulate the growth and development of muscle tissue, leading to increased strength and size. When you stop exercising, the stimulus for muscle growth diminishes, and the muscle may gradually decrease in size or atrophy (break down).

- Fat Tissue: Fat tissue, on the other hand, serves as an energy storage system in the body. It consists of adipocytes, which store excess energy in the form of triglycerides. When energy intake exceeds expenditure, fat cells enlarge, leading to an increase in body fat percentage. Conversely, when there is an energy deficit, the body may utilize stored fat for energy.

3. Factors Influencing Muscle and Fat Changes:

- Exercise: Regular resistance training and physical activity play a crucial role in maintaining and building muscle mass. When exercise is reduced or discontinued, muscle tissue may undergo changes due to decreased stimulation.

- Caloric Balance: Caloric intake and expenditure significantly impact body composition. Consuming excess calories without sufficient physical activity can lead to fat accumulation. Conversely, creating a calorie deficit through proper nutrition and exercise promotes fat loss.

- Aging and Hormonal Changes: Aging and hormonal fluctuations can affect muscle and fat distribution. As individuals age, muscle mass tends to naturally decrease, while fat accumulation may increase if dietary habits and exercise routines remain unchanged.

Understanding the distinction between muscle and fat is essential for debunking the myth that muscle can turn into fat. When you stop exercising, muscle tissue may decrease in size or atrophy due to reduced stimulation, while fat accumulation can occur if calorie intake exceeds expenditure.

If you take time off and notice your physique appears smaller or flatter, it is most likely due to glycogen loss, not actual muscle loss (atrophy). Glycogen and hydration levels will return to normal very quickly as soon as you begin to refuel and rehydrate again. But if you have been inactive for longer than 3 weeks, your muscle may start to break down and you might lose real muscle mass.

Starvation Mode

Starvation mode is a commonly misunderstood concept in the realm of weight loss and metabolism. Many people believe that drastically reducing calorie intake leads to the body entering a state of "starvation mode," where the metabolism slows down and weight loss becomes difficult or impossible. However, it's important to debunk this myth and provide a clear understanding of how the body actually responds to calorie restriction.

The notion of starvation mode suggests that when you significantly decrease your calorie intake, your body perceives it as a threat and adapts by conserving energy. It is believed that this adaptive response includes a reduction in metabolic rate, making it harder to lose weight. While it may seem logical, the reality is quite different.

In reality, the human body is a remarkable machine designed to survive and adapt to changing circumstances. When you reduce your calorie intake, the body responds by adjusting its energy expenditure to maintain balance. It does this through a process called metabolic adaptation, where the metabolic rate may slightly decrease, but not to the extent that it sabotages weight loss efforts.

The extent of metabolic adaptation is often exaggerated, especially in relation to modest calorie deficits. While it is true that prolonged severe calorie restriction can lead to metabolic changes, the average person who follows a sensible, moderate calorie deficit for weight loss will not experience the drastic slowdown of their metabolism.

In fact, when you create a calorie deficit through a balanced and sustainable approach, your body taps into its energy stores, primarily fat, to make up for the shortfall. This results in weight loss. The key is to maintain a moderate calorie deficit, which is typically recommended to be around 500 calories per day, depending on individual factors such as body weight, activity level, and goals.

It's important to note that weight loss is not solely about calories in versus calories out. Factors such as the quality of the food you consume, macronutrient distribution, and overall lifestyle habits play significant roles in your body's response to a calorie deficit.

Rather than worrying about triggering a mythical starvation mode, focus on adopting a well-rounded approach to weight loss that includes a balanced, nutrient-dense diet, regular physical activity, and mindful eating habits. These strategies promote sustainable weight loss, support metabolic health, and contribute to overall well-being.

The body is adaptable and resilient. By creating a modest calorie deficit and making healthy lifestyle choices, you can achieve weight loss without the fear of entering a non-existent starvation mode. Focus on long-term sustainability, nourishing your body, and making positive changes that promote overall health and well-being.

All Fats Are Bad

The belief that all fats are bad for your health is a common misconception that has misled many people on their nutritional journey. It's time to set the record straight and shed light on the importance of healthy fats in your diet.

Not all fats are created equal. While it's true that certain fats, such as trans fats and excessive saturated fats, can have negative effects on health when consumed in large amounts, it's crucial to understand that there are also fats that are beneficial and essential for optimal well-being.

Healthy fats, also known as unsaturated fats, play a vital role in various bodily functions and can offer numerous health benefits. These fats are typically found in plant-based sources such as avocados, nuts, seeds, and oils like olive oil, as well as in fatty fish like salmon and tuna.

Healthy fats provide a concentrated source of energy, help the body absorb fat-soluble vitamins (A, D, E, and K), and support the production of essential hormones. They also contribute to satiety, keeping you feeling full and satisfied after meals, which can be beneficial for weight management.

Moreover, healthy fats are crucial for heart health. They can help lower bad cholesterol levels (LDL) and increase good cholesterol levels (HDL), thereby reducing the risk of heart disease and stroke. Consuming moderate amounts of healthy fats as part of a balanced diet has been associated with improved cardiovascular health.

Incorporating sources of healthy fats into your meals and snacks can be enjoyable and nourishing. Add slices of avocado to your salads, sprinkle a handful of nuts or seeds on your yogurt or oatmeal, drizzle olive oil over roasted vegetables, or enjoy a serving of fatty fish a couple of times per week.

It's important to remember that while healthy fats are beneficial, moderation is key. Fats, regardless of their type, are calorie-dense, so it's essential to consume them in appropriate portions to maintain a balanced and healthy diet.

By embracing healthy fats and incorporating them into your eating habits, you can improve the nutritional quality of your diet, support overall health, and enjoy a wide range of delicious and satisfying foods. Remember, not all fats are bad, and including the right fats in your diet can be a step toward achieving optimal well-being.

Supplements For Quick Fixes

In the quest for better health and fitness, it's common to come across enticing promises of quick fixes and miraculous results offered by various supplements. However, it's essential to address the misconception that supplements alone can transform your body without the foundation of proper nutrition, exercise, and sleep.

While certain supplements can play a supportive role in achieving your health and fitness goals, it's important to remember that they are not magic potions that can replace a well-rounded approach. Supplements should be viewed as additions to an already solid foundation of healthy lifestyle habits rather than standalone solutions.

Proper nutrition and exercise are the cornerstones of any successful health and fitness journey. Without a well-balanced diet that provides essential nutrients and supports overall health, no supplement can truly deliver the desired results. Similarly, exercise is crucial for building strength, endurance, and maintaining a healthy body composition.

Supplements can be beneficial in certain cases to fill in specific nutrient gaps or support specific goals. For example, protein powders can be useful for individuals who struggle to meet their protein needs through food alone or for convenient post-workout recovery. Similarly, certain vitamins and minerals may require supplementation for individuals with specific deficiencies.

However, it's important to approach supplements with caution and proper knowledge. Not all supplements are created equal, and their efficacy and safety can vary. It's advisable to consult with a healthcare professional or registered dietitian before adding any supplements to your regimen.

Remember, no supplement can replace the power of a nutritious and well-balanced diet, regular physical activity, and consistent lifestyle habits. It's the combination of these factors that lays the foundation for long-term success and sustainable results.

Rather than relying solely on supplements, prioritize a whole-foods-based diet that includes a variety of nutrient-dense foods, such as fruits, vegetables, lean proteins, whole grains, and healthy fats. Combine this with regular exercise, including both cardiovascular and strength training activities, to promote overall health, strength, and vitality.

By focusing on building a strong foundation of healthy habits and utilizing supplements as appropriate additions, you can optimize your journey toward improved health and fitness. Emphasize the importance of a well-rounded approach, and remember that sustainable and lasting results are achieved through consistent effort, patience, and a holistic approach to your overall well-being.

High Rep Ranges Tone Your Muscles & Low Rep Ranges Make You Bulky

One prevailing myth in the realm of fitness is the idea that using high rep ranges will make your muscles more defined, while low rep ranges will make you bulky. This misconception can lead to confusion and improper training approaches. Let's bust this myth and shed light on the truth behind rep ranges and muscle definition.

Muscle definition is primarily determined by two key factors: body fat percentage and muscle size. To achieve a more defined look, it's essential to focus on reducing body fat while maintaining or building lean muscle mass. Rep ranges alone do not dictate whether you'll achieve a defined or bulky physique.

High rep ranges, typically considered to be around 12-15 repetitions or more, are often associated with muscular endurance and can be effective for improving cardiovascular fitness and endurance capacity. While high reps can provide a challenging workout and increase muscular endurance, they don't inherently lead to increased muscle definition on their own.

On the other hand, low rep ranges, typically ranging from 1-6 repetitions, are often associated with strength and power training. Contrary to popular belief, lifting heavy weights in low rep ranges does not automatically make you bulky. Building significant muscle mass requires a combination of factors, including progressive overload, proper nutrition, and adequate recovery. It's important to note that building bulky muscles is a deliberate process that involves specific training protocols, nutrition plans, and sometimes even genetic factors.

To achieve muscle definition, regardless of rep range, it's crucial to focus on a few key principles:

1. Progressive overload: Consistently challenging your muscles by gradually increasing the resistance or intensity over time. This can be achieved through a variety of rep ranges and training techniques.

2. Proper nutrition: Maintaining a well-balanced diet that supports muscle development and promotes a healthy body composition. This includes consuming adequate protein, carbohydrates, and healthy fats.

3. Body fat management: Lowering overall body fat percentage through a combination of proper nutrition, regular exercise, and a healthy lifestyle. This is crucial for enhancing muscle definition and showcasing the underlying muscle tone.

4. Varied training approaches: Incorporating a mix of rep ranges, training modalities, and exercises to stimulate different muscle fibers and promote overall muscle development.

Remember, there is no one-size-fits-all approach to training, and individual responses can vary. Instead of fixating solely on rep ranges, focus on developing a well-rounded training program that includes a mix of rep ranges, compound exercises, isolation exercises, and appropriate rest periods. This approach ensures that you target different aspects of muscle development, strength, endurance, and overall fitness.

Ultimately, achieving muscle definition is a multifaceted process that involves a combination of factors, including proper nutrition, consistent training, and body fat management. By adopting a holistic approach and dispelling the myth that rep ranges alone dictate muscle definition, you can work towards your goals with a clearer understanding and more effective strategies.

Cardio Kills Gains

One common myth that deserves debunking is the belief that cardio kills gains. Many individuals fear that engaging in cardiovascular exercise will hinder their muscle-building progress. While there is some truth to this misconception, it's important to understand the underlying factors at play.

The idea that cardio can impede muscle gains stems from the notion that excessive cardiovascular exercise can lead to an increased calorie expenditure. When combined with insufficient calorie intake, this can create an energy deficit that may negatively impact muscle growth. However, it's essential to recognize that it's not the cardio itself that directly hampers gains, but rather the inadequate nutrition accompanying it.

Additionally, the timing of cardio in relation to resistance training can influence its impact on muscle growth. If cardio is performed before resistance training, it can pre-fatigue the body, potentially compromising strength and performance during weightlifting exercises. This can result in suboptimal muscle stimulation and limit potential gains. However, it's important to note that performing cardio after resistance training or on separate days can mitigate these concerns, allowing for optimal recovery and muscle-building stimulus during weightlifting sessions.

The key takeaway is that cardio, when properly integrated into a well-designed training and nutrition plan, can coexist with muscle growth goals. By ensuring sufficient calorie intake and appropriately timing cardio sessions, individuals can reap the cardiovascular benefits without compromising their muscle-building endeavors. It's crucial to prioritize proper nutrition, providing the body with the necessary fuel to support both muscle growth and cardiovascular health. Remember, it's the combination of a well-rounded fitness approach and balanced nutrition that yields the best results in achieving your goals.

Lifting Weights Stunts Growth

One prevalent myth that needs to be dispelled is the belief that lifting weights stunts growth, particularly in adolescents. This misconception has discouraged many individuals, especially young people, from engaging in resistance training out of fear that it may hinder their growth and development. However, it's important to separate fact from fiction and understand the actual impact of weightlifting on growth.

The idea that weightlifting stunts growth primarily stems from concerns over potential injuries that can occur when lifting weights improperly or with excessive loads. Injuries sustained during weightlifting, especially to the growth plates, can interfere with proper growth and development. However, it's crucial to note that when performed with appropriate technique, proper supervision, and appropriate loads, weightlifting can have numerous benefits for growth and development.

In fact, resistance training and weightlifting can stimulate the production of growth hormone and testosterone, two key hormones involved in growth and muscle development. These hormones play crucial roles in the body's ability to repair and build new tissues, including muscle and bone. Engaging in resistance training can help optimize the secretion of these hormones, promoting healthy growth and development.

Moreover, weightlifting can have a positive impact on bone health, increasing bone mineral density and strength. This can be particularly beneficial during adolescence, a critical period for bone development. By engaging in weightlifting and resistance training, individuals can promote optimal bone growth, reduce the risk of osteoporosis later in life, and support overall skeletal health.

It's important to emphasize that weightlifting, like any form of physical activity, should be approached with proper form, technique, and supervision. This applies especially to young individuals who are still growing. By adhering to safe practices and gradually progressing the intensity and load of the exercises, the risk of injuries can be minimized, allowing individuals to safely reap the benefits of weightlifting and resistance training for their growth and development.

In conclusion, weightlifting does not stunt growth when performed with proper technique, supervision, and appropriate loads. In fact, it can trigger the release of growth hormone and testosterone, promoting healthy growth, muscle development, and bone strength. By adopting safe practices and seeking guidance from qualified professionals, individuals can enjoy the numerous benefits that resistance training and weightlifting offer without compromising their growth and development.

VII: Flexibility & Mobility

The Importance Of Flexibility & Mobility

Flexibility and mobility are often overlooked aspects of fitness, but they play a vital role in optimizing your physical performance and overall well-being. These two key components are essential for maintaining joint health, preventing injuries, and enhancing your body's movement quality.

One of the primary benefits of flexibility and mobility is the prevention of injuries. When your muscles and joints are flexible and mobile, they are less prone to strains, sprains, and other musculoskeletal injuries. By maintaining adequate range of motion, you reduce the likelihood of compensatory movements and imbalances that can lead to overuse injuries.

Flexibility and mobility also play a crucial role in enhancing athletic performance. Whether you're an elite athlete or a recreational fitness enthusiast, having optimal range of motion and joint mobility allows you to perform movements with greater efficiency and effectiveness. It can enhance your speed, power, agility, and coordination, enabling you to excel in various physical activities.

Moreover, flexibility and mobility contribute to the overall quality of your movement patterns. When your body can move freely and without restrictions, you experience better biomechanics and motor control. This translates into improved posture, balance, and body alignment, which are essential for proper movement execution and injury prevention.

Additionally, flexibility and mobility are vital for joint health and longevity. As we age, our joints naturally undergo wear and tear, which can lead to stiffness and decreased range of motion. By maintaining and improving flexibility and mobility, you can counteract these effects, preserving joint health and minimizing the risk of age-related conditions such as arthritis.

Remember to listen to your body and progress gradually. Not everyone starts at the same level, and it's important to respect your current limitations while gradually expanding your range of motion. Over time, with consistent practice, you'll notice improvements in your flexibility and mobility, leading to enhanced physical performance and overall well-being.

The Difference Between Flexibility and Mobility

Flexibility and mobility are two terms commonly used in the realm of movement and fitness, but they represent distinct aspects of our physical capabilities. Understanding the difference between these concepts can help us develop a more comprehensive approach to optimizing our body's potential.

Flexibility refers to the range of motion of a muscle or joint. It is the ability of a muscle or group of muscles to lengthen and stretch, allowing for movement across a joint. When we talk about flexibility, we are essentially assessing how far a muscle or joint can be stretched or extended.

On the other hand, mobility encompasses not only flexibility but also the ability to move a joint actively through its full range of motion. It involves joint stability, control, and the integration of multiple muscle groups to execute a movement smoothly. Mobility is about how well we can actively control and perform movements with the available range of motion.

To put it simply, flexibility is a passive characteristic, while mobility is an active one. Flexibility refers to the potential range of motion a muscle or joint can achieve, whereas mobility reflects how well we can use that range of motion in functional activities and movements.

For example, consider a person with excellent flexibility in their hamstrings. They can easily touch their toes while keeping their legs straight. This showcases their hamstring's flexibility. However, mobility comes into play when they actively engage their hamstrings to perform a movement like a deep squat. Mobility involves not only having flexible hamstrings but also utilizing that flexibility in functional movements.

Having a good balance of both flexibility and mobility is essential for optimal movement patterns, injury prevention, and performance. While flexibility allows for a greater range of motion, mobility ensures that we can control and utilize that range effectively.

To enhance flexibility, passive stretching techniques like static stretching or using tools like foam rollers can be beneficial. These methods aim to increase the extensibility of muscles and connective tissues. On the other hand, improving mobility requires active movements that challenge and strengthen the muscles and joints through their full range of motion. Dynamic stretching, mobility drills, and functional exercises can help improve mobility.

By understanding the distinction between flexibility and mobility, we can tailor our training and movement practices accordingly. Assessing and addressing both aspects in our fitness routines can lead to improved movement quality, reduced risk of injury, and enhanced performance in various physical activities.

In summary, flexibility relates to the range of motion of a muscle or joint, while mobility encompasses the active control and utilization of that range of motion. Both flexibility and mobility are vital for optimal movement patterns and overall physical well-being. By nurturing both aspects, we can unlock our body's potential for greater functional capabilities and enjoy a more active and fulfilling lifestyle.

The Benefits Of Flexibility & Mobility Training

Flexibility and mobility training may not always receive the same level of attention as strength or cardiovascular exercises, but their importance should not be overlooked. Incorporating regular flexibility and mobility exercises into your fitness routine can bring about a multitude of benefits that go beyond simply being able to touch your toes or perform deep squats. Let's explore the advantages of prioritizing flexibility and mobility training.

1. Improved Posture: Flexibility and mobility exercises help lengthen tight muscles and release tension, promoting better posture. By enhancing the flexibility of muscles such as the hip flexors, chest, and shoulders, you can counteract the negative effects of prolonged sitting or sedentary lifestyles. Improved posture not only contributes to a more aesthetically pleasing appearance but also reduces the risk of pain or discomfort associated with poor alignment.

2. Enhanced Athletic Performance: Whether you're an athlete or engage in recreational sports and activities, flexibility and mobility play a vital role in optimizing performance. Increased joint range of motion allows for greater movement efficiency, agility, and power. Flexibility in specific muscle groups directly impacts sport-specific movements, such as the ability to reach, stretch, or rotate effectively. By incorporating flexibility and mobility exercises tailored to your activities, you can boost your athletic prowess and take your performance to the next level.

3. Reduced Muscle Soreness: Flexibility and mobility training can help alleviate muscle soreness and tightness following intense workouts. By increasing blood flow to the muscles and enhancing their elasticity, you facilitate the removal of metabolic waste

products and promote faster recovery. Engaging in post-workout stretching or mobility exercises can aid in reducing the stiffness and discomfort commonly experienced after exercise.

4. Injury Prevention: Maintaining adequate flexibility and mobility is crucial for injury prevention. By addressing muscle imbalances, increasing joint range of motion, and promoting proper movement patterns, you can reduce the risk of strains, sprains, and other musculoskeletal injuries. Flexibility and mobility training help optimize biomechanics and ensure that your body can move efficiently and safely during various activities.

5. Enhanced Functional Movement: Flexibility and mobility training improve your ability to perform everyday tasks with ease. From bending down to pick up objects to reaching overhead to perform household chores, having optimal range of motion and mobility in joints allows for fluid, pain-free movement. Flexibility and mobility exercises promote functional movement patterns that translate into improved quality of life and a greater capacity to engage in activities you enjoy.

Incorporating flexibility and mobility exercises into your fitness routine doesn't have to be time-consuming or complicated. Simple stretching routines, mobility drills, yoga, or Pilates sessions can offer significant benefits. Aim to dedicate a few minutes each day to these exercises or integrate them into your warm-up or cool-down routines.

Remember, flexibility and mobility training are not one-time achievements but ongoing processes. Consistency is key to maintaining and improving these aspects of physical fitness. Over time, you'll experience the incremental benefits that flexibility and mobility training bring, leading to a more balanced, resilient, and functional body.

Embrace the power of flexibility and mobility training, and unlock your body's full potential. Enhance your posture, elevate your athletic performance, reduce muscle soreness, prevent injuries, and enjoy the freedom of movement that comes with a flexible and mobile body.

Stretching Techniques

Stretching is an essential component of any well-rounded fitness routine, as it helps improve flexibility, increase joint range of motion, and prepare the body for physical activity. There are various stretching techniques available, each with its unique approach and benefits. Let's explore three popular stretching methods: static stretching, dynamic stretching, and proprioceptive neuromuscular facilitation (PNF) stretching.

1. Static Stretching: Static stretching involves holding a stretch in a comfortable position for a set duration, typically ranging from 15 to 60 seconds. This technique aims to lengthen and relax the target muscles, promoting improved flexibility over time. Static stretching is commonly performed after a workout or during a separate stretching session. It is beneficial for improving overall flexibility and increasing joint range of motion.

To perform static stretching, follow these steps:

- Choose a specific muscle group you want to stretch.

- Assume a position where the muscle is elongated and feel a gentle stretch.

- Hold the stretch without bouncing or forcing the movement.

- Breathe deeply and relax into the stretch, aiming to feel a gentle pull, but not pain or discomfort.

- Hold the stretch for the desired duration and repeat on the opposite side if applicable.

2. Dynamic Stretching: Dynamic stretching involves moving through a controlled range of motion that mimics the movements

of the activity or sport you are about to perform. Unlike static stretching, dynamic stretching is done with fluid movements and no prolonged holds. This technique helps increase blood flow, activate muscles, and enhance flexibility while also preparing the body for physical exertion.

To perform dynamic stretching, follow these steps:

- Choose dynamic exercises that target the muscles you will be using during your activity.

- Perform controlled movements through a full range of motion.

- Start with smaller, controlled movements and gradually increase the intensity and range of motion.

- Perform dynamic stretches for around 10 to 15 repetitions or for a set distance or time.

- Focus on maintaining proper form and control throughout the movements.

3. Proprioceptive Neuromuscular Facilitation (PNF) Stretching: PNF stretching combines passive stretching with muscle contractions to enhance flexibility. It involves contracting and relaxing the muscles being stretched to achieve a deeper stretch. PNF stretching is typically performed with a partner, but self-assisted techniques can also be used.

To perform PNF stretching, follow these steps:

- Assume a stretch position for the target muscle.

- Contract the muscle being stretched against resistance for around 5 to 10 seconds.

- Relax the muscle and move into a deeper stretch while exhaling.

- Hold the deeper stretch for around 15 to 30 seconds.

- Repeat the contract-relax sequence one or two more times, gradually moving into a deeper stretch each time.

When deciding which stretching technique to use, consider the specific needs of your activity or workout. Static stretching is most effective when performed after exercise or during dedicated stretching sessions. Dynamic stretching is ideal for warming up before physical activity, as it prepares the body for movement. PNF stretching can be incorporated to improve flexibility and address specific muscle imbalances.

Remember, proper form and technique are crucial when performing any stretching technique to ensure safety and effectiveness. Always listen to your body and avoid stretching to the point of pain. Consistency and gradual progression are key to achieving long-term flexibility gains.

By incorporating a combination of static stretching, dynamic stretching, and PNF stretching into your fitness routine, you can enhance your flexibility, increase joint range of motion, and optimize your overall performance. Experiment with different techniques, find what works best for you, and enjoy the benefits of a flexible and mobile body.

Joint Mobility Exercises

Joint mobility is essential for maintaining optimal function, preventing injuries, and supporting overall movement quality. Incorporating joint mobility exercises into your fitness routine can help improve joint range of motion, reduce stiffness, and enhance joint stability. Let's explore a range of exercises that target different major joints in the body, allowing you to unlock greater mobility and freedom of movement.

1. Shoulder Circles: Stand tall with your feet shoulder-width apart. Extend your arms out to the sides at shoulder level. Begin by making circular motions with your shoulders, gradually increasing the size of the circles. Perform both clockwise and counterclockwise rotations. This exercise helps improve shoulder mobility and flexibility.

2. Hip Rotations: Stand with your feet hip-width apart. Place your hands on your hips for support. Initiate the movement from your hips and slowly rotate them in a circular motion, first in one direction and then the other. Perform smooth and controlled rotations to improve hip mobility and enhance the range of motion in your hip joints.

3. Spinal Twists: Sit on the floor with your legs extended in front of you. Place your right hand on the floor behind your back for support. Bend your left knee and cross it over your right leg, placing your left foot on the floor next to your right knee. Gently twist your torso to the left, using your left hand to assist the rotation. Hold the stretch for a few seconds, then repeat on the other side. Spinal twists help increase mobility in the thoracic spine and promote better spinal rotation.

4. Ankle Circles: Sit on a chair or the floor with your legs extended in front of you. Lift one foot off the ground and rotate your ankle in a circular motion. Perform several rotations in one direction, then switch to the opposite direction. Repeat with the other foot. Ankle circles enhance ankle mobility, which is important for activities that involve walking, running, and jumping.

5. Wrist Flexion and Extension: Extend one arm in front of you with your palm facing down. Use your other hand to gently pull your fingers backward, stretching your wrist and forearm. Hold the stretch for a few seconds, then switch to the other hand. Next, flip your hand, so your palm is facing up, and gently pull your fingers downward to stretch the opposite side of your wrist and forearm. This exercise helps improve wrist mobility and flexibility.

Remember, these exercises are just a starting point. It's important to address all major joints in the body, including the shoulders, hips, spine, ankles, wrists, and others. Incorporate a variety of joint mobility exercises that target different areas to ensure comprehensive joint health and functionality.

Perform these exercises in a controlled manner, paying attention to proper form and avoiding any pain or discomfort. Start with gentle movements and gradually increase the range of motion as your joints become more mobile and flexible. Consistency is key, so aim to include joint mobility exercises in your regular fitness routine to maintain and enhance your joint health over time.

By incorporating joint mobility exercises into your fitness regimen, you can unlock greater freedom of movement, enhance joint range of motion, and promote overall joint health.

Flexibility Training For Specific Muscle Groups

Flexibility training plays a crucial role in maintaining balanced muscle function, preventing injuries, and enhancing overall physical performance. By targeting specific muscle groups with stretching exercises, you can improve muscle flexibility, reduce muscle imbalances, and promote better posture. Let's explore stretches for major muscle groups to help you unleash your range of motion.

1. Hamstring Stretch: Sit on the floor with one leg extended in front of you and the other leg bent, with the sole of your foot touching your inner thigh. Keeping your back straight, reach forward toward your toes, aiming to feel a gentle stretch in the back of your thigh. Hold the stretch for 20 to 30 seconds on each side.

2. Quadriceps Stretch: Stand tall and grab your ankle or foot behind you. Gently pull your heel toward your glutes, feeling a stretch in the front of your thigh. Keep your knees close together and your torso upright. Hold the stretch for 20 to 30 seconds on each leg.

3. Chest Stretch: Stand near a wall or doorway. Extend one arm to the side, placing your hand on the wall or frame. Slowly rotate your body away from the extended arm, feeling a stretch across your chest. Hold the stretch for 20 to 30 seconds on each side.

4. Back Stretch: Lie on your back and hug your knees into your chest. Rock gently from side to side to release tension in your lower back. For a deeper stretch, you can extend one leg straight while keeping the other knee hugged to your chest. Hold the stretch for 20 to 30 seconds on each side.

5. Shoulder Stretch: Stand tall and place one arm across your chest, using your other arm to gently pull the extended arm closer to your body. Feel the stretch in your shoulder and the back of your arm. Hold the stretch for 20 to 30 seconds on each side.

6. Calf Stretch: Stand facing a wall, placing both hands on the wall at shoulder height. Step one foot back, keeping the heel flat on the ground. Lean forward, feeling the stretch in your calf muscle. Hold the stretch for 20 to 30 seconds on each leg.

Remember, when performing these stretches, it's important to maintain proper form and technique. Avoid bouncing or jerking movements, and breathe deeply to relax into each stretch. Aim for a gentle, comfortable stretch without pushing yourself to the point of pain.

Flexibility training is most effective when done regularly and consistently. Incorporate these stretches into your fitness routine, aiming to stretch major muscle groups at least two to three times per week. As you progress, you may find that you can increase the duration of each stretch or explore more advanced variations.

By targeting specific muscle groups with focused stretches, you can improve flexibility, enhance muscle balance, and promote better movement quality. Embrace the benefits of increased range of motion and enjoy the freedom of flexible muscles as you engage in various physical activities.

Remember, flexibility training should be complemented by other components of fitness, such as strength training and cardiovascular exercise, to achieve a well-rounded fitness routine. Listen to your body, respect your limitations, and gradually work towards greater flexibility and mobility.

Incorporating Flexibility & Mobility Into Workouts

Flexibility and mobility exercises are not standalone activities; they are integral components of a well-rounded workout routine. By incorporating these exercises strategically, you can enhance your performance, reduce the risk of injuries, and promote better recovery. Let's explore how you can integrate flexibility and mobility into different parts of your workouts.

1. Warm-Up Routine: Begin your workouts with a dynamic warm-up that includes mobility exercises. Perform movements that mimic the exercises you'll be doing during your main workout, but at a lower intensity. For example, if your workout involves squats, include bodyweight squats or leg swings to warm up your hips and lower body. This helps to activate the muscles, increase blood flow, and prepare your body for the upcoming movements.

2. Active Rest Periods: Instead of completely resting between sets of strength exercises, utilize your rest periods for mobility exercises. Perform dynamic stretches or mobility drills that target the muscle groups you are training. For instance, if you're focusing on upper body exercises, incorporate shoulder circles or arm swings during your rest breaks. This not only improves flexibility but also helps to maintain your heart rate and keeps your body warm throughout the workout.

3. Cool-Down Routine: At the end of your workout, include static stretches and deeper mobility exercises in your cool-down routine. Focus on the major muscle groups you engaged during your workout. Hold each stretch for 20 to 30 seconds, aiming for a gentle stretch without overexerting yourself. This allows your muscles to relax and

lengthen, promoting better recovery and reducing post-workout muscle soreness.

4. Recovery Days: On your recovery or active rest days, dedicate some time to dedicated flexibility and mobility sessions. Use this opportunity to work on specific areas of tightness or limited mobility. Explore various stretching techniques, such as static stretching, dynamic stretching, or proprioceptive neuromuscular facilitation (PNF) stretching, to target different muscle groups and improve range of motion.

Remember, flexibility and mobility exercises should be performed with proper form and technique. Focus on quality of movement rather than quantity, and listen to your body's feedback. Avoid pushing yourself into painful or uncomfortable positions and make gradual progress over time.

By incorporating flexibility and mobility exercises into your workouts, you not only improve your joint health, but you also enhance your overall movement quality and performance. These exercises help to correct muscle imbalances, improve posture, and reduce the risk of injuries during training. Additionally, they promote better recovery, allowing your muscles to adapt and grow stronger.

Whether you're engaged in strength training, cardiovascular workouts, or any other physical activities, integrating flexibility and mobility exercises into your routine will unlock your body's full potential. Embrace the benefits of increased range of motion, improved muscle function, and enhanced overall fitness. Your body will thank you for the investment in its longevity and well-being.

Frequency and Progression

When it comes to flexibility and mobility training, consistency and progressive overload are key. To achieve noticeable improvements in your flexibility and range of motion, it's essential to establish a regular training routine and gradually challenge your body to adapt. Let's delve into the concepts of frequency and progression in flexibility and mobility training.

1. Frequency of Training: Aim to incorporate flexibility and mobility exercises into your weekly workout routine at least two to three times per week. Consistency is crucial for making meaningful changes in your flexibility. Regular training sessions allow your body to adapt and gradually increase its range of motion. However, be mindful not to overdo it—giving your muscles time to recover is just as important.

2. Duration of Sessions: The duration of each flexibility and mobility session will depend on your individual needs and time availability. A typical session can range from 10 to 30 minutes. Remember, quality matters more than quantity. Focus on performing each stretch or mobility exercise with proper form and control, emphasizing the target muscle group and range of motion.

3. Progressive Overload: Like any other form of training, progression is crucial in flexibility and mobility work. Start with stretches and exercises that are challenging but manageable, avoiding any pain. As your body adapts and becomes more flexible, gradually increase the intensity or range of motion. This can be done by holding stretches for a longer duration, reaching further in a range of motion, or incorporating more advanced mobility exercises.

4. Listen to Your Body: Pay close attention to how your body responds to each stretch or mobility exercise. Avoid forcing movements or pushing through pain. It's important to distinguish between discomfort associated with stretching and actual pain from improper form or overstretching. Respect your body's limitations and progress at a pace that feels comfortable and safe.

5. Incorporate Variety: Keep your flexibility and mobility routine engaging and effective by incorporating a variety of stretches and exercises. Target different muscle groups and explore different stretching techniques, such as static, dynamic, and PNF stretching. This helps to ensure balanced flexibility throughout your body and prevents muscle imbalances or overuse injuries.

6. Individualize Your Approach: Remember that everyone's flexibility and mobility levels are unique. Modify stretches and exercises to suit your own body and limitations. You may need to adjust the duration, range of motion, or intensity of each exercise to best accommodate your current abilities and goals.

By training with the right frequency and gradually progressing over time, you'll witness improvements in your flexibility and mobility. Increased range of motion not only enhances your performance in various physical activities but also promotes better posture, joint health, and overall movement quality.

Consistency, patience, and dedication are key to long-term success in flexibility and mobility training. As you progress, celebrate each milestone and continue challenging yourself to reach new levels of flexibility and range of motion.

VIII: Goal Setting & Progress Tracking

The importance of setting specific, measurable, achievable, relevant, and time-bound (SMART) goals cannot be overstated when it comes to personal development, growth, and success. SMART goals provide a clear framework and roadmap for achieving desired outcomes, whether it's in fitness, career, relationships, or any other area of life.

1. Specific: Setting specific goals means clearly defining what you want to achieve. It involves answering the questions of who, what, where, when, why, and how. The more specific your goal, the better you can focus your efforts and resources towards its attainment.

2. Measurable: Measurable goals allow you to track your progress and determine whether you are moving in the right direction. By establishing concrete criteria for success, such as quantifiable metrics or milestones, you can objectively assess your performance and make adjustments if necessary.

3. Achievable: Goals should be challenging yet attainable. It's important to set realistic targets that stretch your capabilities but are within your reach. This helps maintain motivation and prevents feelings of overwhelm or discouragement. Breaking larger goals into smaller, manageable steps can make them more achievable.

4. Relevant: Goals should align with your overall vision, values, and aspirations. They should be meaningful and relevant to your life's purpose. By setting goals that are personally significant, you are more likely to stay committed and inspired throughout the journey.

5. Time-bound: Setting a specific timeframe or deadline creates a sense of urgency and accountability. It helps you prioritize your actions and allocate resources effectively. Having a clear endpoint

also allows for reflection, evaluation, and adjustment of strategies as needed.

6. Create A Plan: Almost every person has goals and desires, but hardly anybody has a plan on how they will achieve these goals and desires. Create a clear and realistic plan on what you will do and how you will do it to achieve your goals. Nothing comes to you by accident, you need to work hard and do what's necessary to get what you want.

7. Focus on The Lead Measures (Actions and Habits) Instead of The Goals: The person who loves and focuses on the journey will come longer than the person who loves and focuses on the destination. Create sustainable habits that lead you towards achieving your goals. E.g. if you want to run 7km in 30 min, set a goal to run 3-5 times a week and progress with an amount of seconds each session.

By following the SMART framework, you increase the likelihood of success in reaching your goals. It provides structure, clarity, and focus, enabling you to measure progress, stay motivated, and make informed decisions along the way.

Remember, setting SMART goals is not a one-time activity. It's an ongoing process of evaluation, adjustment, and setting new targets as you progress. Regularly reviewing and refining your goals ensures that they remain relevant and aligned with your evolving needs and aspirations.

In conclusion, incorporating SMART goal-setting principles into your life empowers you to take charge of your destiny and achieve meaningful outcomes. Whether you're striving for personal growth, career advancement, or overall well-being, SMART goals serve as a powerful tool to turn aspirations into reality.

Strategies for Tracking Progress and Reaching Your Goals

Strategies for tracking progress and staying motivated are crucial for maintaining momentum and achieving long-term success in any endeavor. While motivation can be a powerful driving force, it can also be fleeting and unreliable. That's why it's important to shift the focus from relying solely on motivation and instead cultivate self-discipline to stay committed even when motivation wanes.

1. Tracking Progress:

- Use a journal or tracking app to record your activities, achievements, and setbacks. This provides a visual representation of your progress, allowing you to see how far you've come and what you need to do to progress further.

- Set specific milestones or markers along the way to track incremental progress. Celebrate each small win, as it reinforces positive behavior and keeps you motivated.

- Regularly assess and evaluate your progress against your goals. This helps identify areas for improvement and adjust your strategies as needed.

2. Goal Visualization:

- Visualize your desired outcome and the benefits it will bring. Create a clear mental image of what success looks like to help keep your motivation alive.

- Use vision boards or other visual tools to display images and words that represent your goals. Surrounding yourself with visual reminders can reinforce your motivation.

3. Accountability:

- Share your goals with a trusted friend, family member, or mentor. Having someone who can hold you accountable can help keep you on track and provide support during challenging times.

- Join a group or community of like-minded individuals working towards similar goals. Engaging with others who share your aspirations can provide motivation, inspiration, and a sense of brotherhood. If you surround yourself with losers, you're more likely to be a loser. If you surround yourself with ambitious and disciplined people who achieve their goals, you're more likely to be a winner.

4. Break Goals into Smaller Steps:

- Divide your larger goals into smaller, actionable steps. This makes them more manageable and allows for a sense of progress and accomplishment along the way.

- Focus on one step at a time, maintaining clarity and direction. Small victories build momentum and confidence, keeping you motivated to continue.

5. Build Self-Discipline:

- Cultivate self-discipline as a foundation for consistent action, even when motivation wavers. Understand that discipline is more reliable and sustainable than relying solely on motivation.

- Develop a routine or schedule that incorporates your goals and desired actions. Make them non-negotiable commitments to yourself, reinforcing the habit of discipline.

6. Embrace the Process:

- Shift your mindset from solely outcome-focused to appreciating the journey and the growth it brings. Recognize that progress takes time and that setbacks are learning opportunities.

- Find joy and fulfillment in the process itself, rather than solely fixating on the end result. Embrace the challenges and lessons that come along the way.

Tracking progress and staying motivated are essential for long-term success. While motivation can provide an initial spark, it's the cultivation of self-discipline and consistent action that sustains progress. By implementing strategies for tracking progress, visualizing goals, cultivating accountability, breaking goals into smaller steps, building self-discipline, and embracing the process, you can stay motivated and achieve your desired outcomes. Remember, success is not just about motivation; it's about consistent effort and disciplined action, even when motivation wavers.

Never, ever rely solely on motivation.

Accountability and Support Systems

Achieving your goals requires more than just individual effort and willpower. It often involves external factors that can provide valuable support and accountability along the way. Accountability and support systems play a crucial role in helping you stay focused, motivated, and consistent in your pursuit of success.

1. Accountability:

Accountability refers to the sense of responsibility and answerability to oneself or others. When you hold yourself accountable, you are more likely to take ownership of your actions and follow through with your commitments. Here's how accountability can positively impact your goal accomplishment:

a. Clear Commitments: By setting clear, specific goals and sharing them with others, you create a sense of responsibility to honor your commitments.

b. Motivation and Focus: Knowing that you are accountable to someone else can boost your motivation and help you stay focused on your goals, even during challenging times.

c. Progress Tracking: Accountability systems often involve regular check-ins or progress updates, allowing you to track your progress and make adjustments as needed.

d. External Feedback and Support: Being accountable to others provides an opportunity to receive valuable feedback, encouragement, and support along your journey.

2. Support Systems:

Support systems are the networks, communities, or individuals who provide guidance, encouragement, and assistance throughout your goal pursuit. Here's why having a strong support system is essential:

a. Emotional Support: Surrounding yourself with like-minded individuals or mentors who understand your aspirations can provide emotional support when facing obstacles or setbacks.

b. Knowledge and Resources: Support systems often offer access to valuable knowledge, expertise, and resources that can enhance your understanding and skill development.

c. Collaboration and Accountability Partners: Engaging with individuals who share similar goals or interests allows for collaboration, idea sharing, and the opportunity to hold each other accountable.

d. Celebration and Recognition: Your support system can celebrate your milestones and achievements, providing positive reinforcement and boosting your confidence.

3. Building Self-Discipline:

While accountability and support systems are beneficial, the most important part is to cultivate self-discipline. Self-discipline involves cultivating habits and routines that align with your goals, even when motivation wanes. Here's why self-discipline matters:

a. Consistency: Self-discipline helps you maintain consistency in your actions, ensuring that you make progress towards your goals even on days when external support or motivation isn't there.

b. Long-term Success: Relying solely on external motivation can be unpredictable. Self-discipline allows you to stay committed and persevere in the absence of external influences.

c. Personal Empowerment: Building self-discipline empowers you to take control of your actions and choices, reducing reliance on external factors for motivation.

In conclusion, accountability and support systems provide valuable assistance in achieving your goals. They offer external motivation, guidance, and feedback, while also fostering self-discipline and personal growth. Embrace accountability, seek out a supportive network, and cultivate self-discipline to create a strong foundation for success. Remember, achieving your goals is a journey, and having the right systems in place can significantly enhance your chances of reaching your desired outcomes.

How To Adjust Your Training & Nutrition Plan Based On Your Progress

As you work towards your goals, it's important to regularly assess your progress and make necessary adjustments to your training and nutrition plan. Adapting your approach based on how your body responds can optimize your results and keep you on the path to success. Here are some key considerations for adjusting your plan:

1. Tracking Progress:

Consistently tracking your progress is essential to understanding how your body is responding to your current training and nutrition regimen. Keep a record of relevant data such as body measurements, weight, strength gains, energy levels, and overall performance.

2. Assessing Results:

Regularly evaluate your progress to determine if you're moving closer to your goals. Look for indicators such as improvements in strength, endurance, body composition, and overall well-being. Consider using tools like body fat calipers, fitness assessments, and performance tests to get a more comprehensive picture of your progress.

3. Training Adjustments:

a. Progressive Overload: If you've reached a plateau in your strength or muscle gains, it may be time to change something in your training or/and nutrition plan. Increase the intensity, volume, or complexity of your workouts gradually to continue challenging your body.

b. Exercise Variation: In general, you should not switch up your exercises frequently. If you keep making progress in your training, keep the same exercise selection and only consider switching it up when you hit a plateau or find a better exercise. There's no such thing as "shocking the muscles". Your muscles react to progressive overload and that's it.

c. Training Frequency: Adjust the frequency of your workouts based on your recovery capacity and progress. You may increase or decrease the number of training sessions per week to optimize recovery and adaptation.

4. Nutrition Adjustments:

a. Caloric Intake: Monitor your body weight and composition regularly. If your goal is fat loss and you've hit a plateau, consider reducing your calorie intake slightly. Conversely, if you're aiming to build muscle and struggling to gain weight, consider increasing your calorie intake.

b. Macronutrient Ratios: Assess the balance of macronutrients (protein, carbohydrates, and fats) in your diet. Adjust the ratios based on your specific goals and individual needs.

c. Nutrient Timing: Pay attention to when you consume your meals and nutrients. Adjust the timing and composition of pre- and post-workout meals to optimize energy levels, recovery, and performance.

5. Recovery and Rest:

Evaluate your recovery and rest practices. If you're experiencing excessive fatigue, poor sleep, or slow recovery between workouts, consider incorporating more rest days or implementing relaxation techniques such as meditation or yoga to promote overall recovery.

6. Seeking Professional Guidance:

If you find it challenging to make appropriate adjustments on your own, consider seeking the guidance of a qualified fitness professional or nutritionist. They can provide personalized recommendations based on your goals, progress, and individual circumstances.

Remember, adjustments to your training and nutrition plan should be based on individual responses and progress. Be patient, listen to your body, and make changes gradually to avoid abrupt disruptions. Regularly reevaluate your plan and be open to experimentation and learning. With a flexible and adaptive approach, you can continuously improve your training & nutrition plans to align with your evolving goals and maximize your results.

IX: Mindset And Motivation

The Importance Of A Positive Mindset & Believing in Yourself

Having a positive mindset and using positive self-talk are crucial elements in achieving your goals. The way you think and talk to yourself greatly influences your actions, emotions, and overall outlook on life. By cultivating a positive mindset and practicing positive self-talk, you can unlock your full potential and overcome obstacles on your journey to success.

One of the key benefits of maintaining a positive mindset is that it helps you stay motivated and focused. When faced with challenges or setbacks, a positive mindset allows you to approach them with resilience and optimism. Instead of dwelling on failures or negative outcomes, you view them as learning opportunities and stepping stones toward growth. With a positive mindset, you believe in your ability to overcome obstacles and keep moving forward.

Positive self-talk is the practice of consciously choosing positive and empowering thoughts and words to guide your inner dialogue. By replacing self-doubt, self-criticism, and negative thoughts with affirmations, encouragement, and constructive self-talk, you create a supportive internal environment. Positive self-talk boosts your self-confidence, enhances your belief in your abilities, and reinforces a positive mindset, even in dark and seemingly hopeless times.

The power of a positive mindset and self-talk extends beyond mere positivity. Research has shown that positive thinking and self-affirmation can improve performance, increase resilience, and enhance overall well-being. When you have a positive mindset, you approach challenges with a solutions-oriented mindset, enabling you to find creative and effective ways to overcome obstacles.

To cultivate a positive mindset and practice positive self-talk, it's important to be mindful of your thoughts and language. Pay attention to the words you use when describing yourself, your progress, and your goals. Replace negative and limiting statements with positive affirmations and constructive thoughts. For example, instead of saying, "I can't do this," replace it with "I am capable of achieving anything I set my mind to."

Additionally, surround yourself with positive influences and supportive individuals who uplift, inspire and hold you accountable. Engage in activities that bring you joy and fulfillment, as they contribute to a positive mindset. Practice gratitude and mindfulness to cultivate a positive perspective on life, you can do this through gratitude journaling (writing down a couple of things you are grateful for, every day) and meditation (there are tons of free apps and videos that guide you through meditation sessions, e.g. Medito).

Remember that building a positive mindset and practicing positive self-talk is a journey that requires consistent effort and self-awareness. Be patient with yourself and celebrate small wins along the way. By adopting a positive mindset and using positive self-talk, you empower yourself to overcome challenges, stay motivated, and ultimately achieve your goals.

Keep believing in yourself, stay positive, and embrace the power of your thoughts and words. You have the ability to create the reality you desire through the lens of a positive mindset and empowering self-talk and beliefs.

Strategies For Staying Motivated and Overcoming Obstacles

Staying motivated and overcoming obstacles are essential components of achieving your goals. It's natural to face challenges and setbacks along your journey, but with the right strategies, you can maintain your motivation and navigate through any obstacles that come your way.

One effective strategy for staying motivated is to clearly define your goals and remind yourself of the reasons why they are important to you. When you have a strong sense of purpose and a clear vision of what you want to achieve, it becomes easier to stay motivated, even when faced with challenges. Write down your goals and keep them visible as a daily reminder of what you're working towards.

Another powerful strategy is to break your goals down into smaller, manageable tasks. By dividing your goals into bite-sized action steps, you can make progress incrementally and celebrate achievements along the way. This approach not only prevents overwhelm but also provides a sense of accomplishment, which fuels your motivation to keep going.

Building a support system is also crucial for staying motivated. Surround yourself with like-minded individuals who share your goals or are supportive of your aspirations. Connect with friends, family, or communities who can provide encouragement, accountability, and guidance. Sharing your journey with others and receiving support can significantly boost your motivation and help you overcome obstacles.

When faced with obstacles, it's important to adopt a growth mindset. View challenges as opportunities for growth and learning rather than as roadblocks. Embrace the belief that setbacks are temporary and that you have the ability to find solutions and grow stronger from them. Cultivate resilience, adaptability, and perseverance as you navigate through obstacles on your path.

Celebrating progress, no matter how small, is an effective strategy to stay motivated. Acknowledge and reward yourself for each milestone achieved. This positive reinforcement not only boosts your motivation but also enhances your self-confidence and belief in your abilities. Take time to reflect on how far you've come and appreciate your efforts and dedication.

Additionally, staying motivated requires self-care and taking care of your overall well-being. Prioritize self-care activities such as exercise, proper nutrition, and sufficient rest. Engage in activities that bring you joy, relaxation, and rejuvenation. When you take care of yourself holistically, you enhance your mental and emotional well-being, which in turn fuels your motivation. Work harder on yourself than you do on your job. - Jim Rohn.

Lastly, it's important to understand that motivation may fluctuate over time. There may be moments when you feel less motivated or encounter periods of stagnation. During these times, focus on building self-discipline rather than relying solely on motivation. Develop habits and routines that support your goals and commit to taking consistent action, even when motivation wavers. It is through consistent effort and self-discipline that you make progress and overcome obstacles.

Remember, staying motivated and overcoming obstacles are ongoing processes. Be patient and kind to yourself throughout your journey. Embrace challenges as opportunities for growth, surround yourself with support, celebrate your progress, and take care of your well-being. With these strategies in place, you can stay motivated and overcome any obstacles that come your way.

Failure is NOT Real

The idea that failure isn't real can be a powerful mindset shift when pursuing your goals and aspirations. Often, we perceive failure as a negative outcome or a setback that signifies the end of our journey. However, reframing our understanding of failure can open up new possibilities and fuel our determination to keep pushing forward.

First and foremost, it's important to recognize that failure is subjective and relative. What may be considered a failure in one context could be seen as a valuable learning experience in another. Instead of viewing setbacks as failures, we can choose to see them as opportunities for growth and development. Each setback or challenge provides valuable lessons and insights that can propel us closer to success.

Embracing the belief that failure doesn't really allow us to detach our self-worth from the outcome of our endeavors. Instead of defining ourselves based on whether we achieve a particular goal or meet certain expectations, we focus on the process and the effort we put in. This mindset shift liberates us from the fear of failure and encourages us to take risks, experiment, and explore new possibilities.

Failure often brings valuable lessons and insights that can lead to breakthroughs and innovation. Many great inventions, discoveries, and achievements were born out of numerous failures and setbacks. By reframing failure as a stepping stone toward success, we can approach challenges with resilience, curiosity, and a growth mindset. We become more open to trying new approaches, adjusting our strategies, and embracing the feedback and lessons learned along the way.

Another important aspect of understanding that failure isn't real is acknowledging that success is almost never a linear path. It's common to encounter obstacles, setbacks, and moments of uncertainty along our journey. These moments are not indications of failure but rather opportunities to reassess, pivot, and evolve. They provide the chance to learn, adapt, and come back stronger than before.

Failure is often intertwined with fear of judgment and perfectionism. By letting go of the notion of failure, we free ourselves from the limitations and expectations imposed by external influences. We allow ourselves to take risks, make mistakes, and pursue our goals with authenticity and courage. This shift in mindset empowers us to embrace vulnerability, learn from our experiences, and grow into our full potential. Remember that the only people that will hate or judge you for failing are the ones who didn't even try, or "failed" and gave up. It never comes from successful people because they know that failure is just another part of your journey to success.

Reframing failure doesn't mean dismissing the emotions that may arise when things don't go as planned. It's natural to feel disappointed, frustrated, or discouraged at times. However, by recognizing that failure is a perception and not an ultimate truth, we can choose how we respond to these emotions. We can use them as fuel to propel us forward, seek support from others, and tap into our resilience and determination.

If you're scared to fail, you might end up not even getting started. When you fail, you get data on what didn't work, which means you become one step closer to accomplishing your goal. The only way to fail is to not do it at all, or give up.

Identity Switch: The Power Of Your Beliefs

Our self-identity plays a crucial role in shaping our thoughts, beliefs, and behaviors. The concept of an "Identity Switch" refers to consciously adopting a new self-identity that aligns with the person we aspire to be. By reframing our self-perception, we can unlock a powerful tool for personal growth and transformation.

The Influence of Self-Identity:

Our self-identity is the narrative we create about ourselves, encompassing our beliefs, values, strengths, and limitations. It forms the foundation of our self-esteem, confidence, and decision-making. When we identify with a particular trait or behavior, it becomes ingrained in our self-concept, guiding our actions and shaping our reality.

The Power of Language:

The language we use to describe ourselves and our goals has a profound impact on our mindset and actions. By shifting our self-talk and using empowering language, we can activate an "Identity Switch" that aligns us with our desired outcomes. For example, instead of saying, "I'm trying to quit smoking," we say, "I don't smoke." This subtle linguistic shift reinforces our new identity and strengthens our commitment to change.

The Role of Beliefs:

Our self-identity is intimately connected to our beliefs. When we believe we are capable, resilient, and worthy of success, we are more likely to take actions that align with those beliefs. By cultivating empowering beliefs about ourselves and our abilities, we can foster a mindset of growth, positivity, and possibility.

Visualizing the Ideal Self:

One powerful technique to facilitate an "Identity Switch" is to visualize our ideal self. By vividly imagining ourselves as the person we aspire to be, we activate the subconscious mind and prime ourselves for success. Through this practice, we create a mental blueprint that guides our thoughts, emotions, and behaviors, ultimately leading us closer to our desired reality.

Embracing Consistency:

Consistency is key in maintaining and reinforcing our new self-identity. By consistently aligning our actions with our desired identity, we create a feedback loop that strengthens our belief in our capabilities. Over time, these aligned actions become habits, solidifying our new identity and making it an integral part of who we are.

Overcoming Limiting Beliefs:

As we embark on our journey of self-identity transformation, it's important to address and overcome any limiting beliefs or self-doubt that may arise. Challenging negative beliefs, seeking support, and cultivating a growth mindset are essential steps in breaking free from self-imposed limitations and fully embracing our new identity. If you say to yourself "You can't do it", then you can't. If you say to yourself "You can do it", you can. It's about believing in yourself.

Living as Your Empowered Self:

The "Identity Switch" is not merely an intellectual exercise but a way of living. As we fully embody our new self-identity, we naturally attract opportunities, people, and experiences that align with our empowered self. We become the architects of our lives, consciously creating a reality that reflects our true potential and aspirations. This might sound pretty weird to some people, but it's almost purely psychological. If you believe something about yourself and it's ingrained in your mind, you start to act like it, even if you're not that person. You have to act a bit delusional. As an example, if you believe you can get girls and that every girl wants you, you will naturally appear more abundant and as if it is actually true.

Our self-identity shapes the trajectory of our lives. By embracing an "Identity Switch" and consciously aligning our thoughts, language, beliefs, and actions with our desired identity, we unlock the transformative power within us. As we embody our empowered self, we create a life of purpose, fulfillment, and limitless possibilities.

Embracing Patience: Finding Joy In The Journey

In our fast-paced and results-driven society, patience has become a rare virtue. However, when it comes to achieving our goals and living a fulfilling life, patience is not only valuable but essential. It is through patience that we can truly embrace and appreciate the journey, finding joy and growth along the way.

The Power of Patience:

Patience is the ability to remain calm, composed, and persistent in the face of challenges and setbacks. It is the understanding that worthwhile accomplishments take time and effort. Patience empowers us to navigate obstacles with grace, maintain a positive mindset, and stay focused on our long-term vision. If you fall in love with patience, you are already closer to succeeding than most people.

Appreciating the Process:

The journey towards our goals is often filled with ups and downs, detours, and unexpected twists. Instead of fixating solely on the end result, cultivating patience allows us to appreciate the process itself. Each step, each small victory, and even each setback becomes an opportunity for growth, learning, and self-discovery.

Finding Joy in the Present:

Impatience often stems from the desire for instant gratification. However, by cultivating patience, we can shift our focus to the present moment and find joy in the here and now. Rather than solely chasing future accomplishments, we learn to savor the journey, celebrating the progress we make each day.

Building Resilience:

Patience acts as a catalyst for building resilience. When we face setbacks or encounter delays, patience allows us to bounce back, reevaluate our approach, and persevere. It helps us maintain a positive outlook, learn from challenges, and adapt our strategies as needed. With patience, we can turn obstacles into stepping stones on our path to success.

Growth and Self-Discovery:

The journey towards our goals is not only about reaching a destination but also about personal growth and self-discovery. Patience allows us to fully immerse ourselves in the process, uncovering our strengths, addressing our weaknesses, and evolving into the best version of ourselves. It is within the journey that we find true transformation.

The Gift of Time:

Patience grants us the gift of time. It gives us the space to reflect, reassess, and make conscious choices. It allows us to make incremental progress, building a solid foundation for lasting success. With patience, we can avoid rushing into impulsive decisions and instead make deliberate choices that align with our values and aspirations. I've heard many people say "It will take too long", and I just thought to myself: the time will go by anyway. Why waste it instead of using it to reach your goals?

Loving the Journey:

When we embrace patience, we learn to love the journey itself. We find beauty in the small victories, appreciate the lessons learned from setbacks, and cherish the personal growth that occurs along the way. We realize that the destination is just one aspect of our journey, and the real joy lies in the experience of becoming who we are meant to be.

Patience is a transformative mindset that allows us to navigate the challenges of life with grace, resilience, and appreciation. By embracing patience and loving the journey, we open ourselves up to profound growth, self-discovery, and joy. As we cultivate patience, we learn to savor each step, celebrate progress, and create a life of fulfillment and purpose.

Mental Health Is Key

In our pursuit of success and happiness, we often overlook the essential element that underpins it all: mental health. Taking care of our mental well-being is not just an optional add-on, but rather a fundamental step towards achieving a fulfilling and balanced life. Recognizing the importance of mental health as the cornerstone of our overall well-being is the first and most crucial step on our journey of self-improvement and personal growth. Having poor mental health means you have it much harder to quit bad habits and addictions, stick to good ones, and even train hard.

The Significance of Mental Health:

Our mental health encompasses our emotional, psychological, and social well-being. It influences how we think, feel, and behave, as well as our ability to handle stress, make decisions, and form healthy relationships. When our mental health is neglected, it can impact every aspect of our lives, including our physical health, productivity, and overall quality of life.

The Role of Mental Health in Achieving Goals:

Prioritizing mental health is the foundation for achieving any goal. Our thoughts, beliefs, and mindset shape our actions and behaviors. When our mental health is compromised, it becomes difficult to stay focused, motivated, and resilient in the face of challenges. By addressing and improving our mental well-being, we create a solid platform from which we can pursue our goals with clarity, determination, and a positive mindset.

Breaking the Stigma:

Society has long perpetuated the stigma surrounding mental health, often viewing it as a sign of weakness or something to be ashamed of. However, we must recognize that mental health is a natural and universal aspect of human existence. Just as we prioritize our physical health, it is essential to treat our mental health with the same level of care, compassion, and understanding.

Building Resilience and Coping Skills:

A healthy mind is resilient and equipped with effective coping mechanisms. When we prioritize our mental health, we develop the necessary tools to navigate life's challenges. We cultivate emotional resilience, learn to manage stress, and develop healthy coping strategies. This resilience empowers us to bounce back from setbacks, maintain balance during difficult times, and adapt to change with greater ease.

Improving Your Mental Health: The most effective way to improve your mental health is simply doing these 4 habits: meditation, sufficient amounts of quality sleep, exercise, and good nutrition. There are many other things you can do as well, but if you do these 4, you're going to get the majority of the benefits out there.

Enhancing Relationships and Connection:

Our mental health significantly influences our relationships and social connections. When we prioritize our mental well-being, we are better equipped to build and nurture healthy relationships. We develop better communication skills, empathy, and emotional intelligence. By fostering positive connections, we create a support system that can uplift us during challenging times and contribute to our overall happiness and wellness.

Creating a Positive Mindset:

A positive mindset is a key ingredient for personal growth and success. By addressing our mental health, we can work on reshaping our thoughts, beliefs, and self-talk. We learn to cultivate self-compassion, challenge negative patterns, and develop a more optimistic outlook. With a positive mindset, we are more open to possibilities, better equipped to handle setbacks, and more motivated to pursue our goals.

By acknowledging the importance of mental well-being as the foundation for a fulfilling life and reaching your goals, you empower yourself to navigate challenges, pursue your goals, and build meaningful connections. By seeing mental health as a top priority, we embark on a transformative journey of self-discovery, personal growth, and ultimately, a life of well-being and purpose.

Visualization & Mental Imagery

Visualization and mental imagery are powerful tools that can significantly impact your journey towards success. By harnessing the power of your mind and imagination, you can enhance your performance, boost your motivation, and manifest your goals into reality.

When you visualize, you create a mental image of yourself accomplishing your desired outcome. It involves vividly imagining the specific details, sensations, and emotions associated with achieving your goals. By repeatedly visualizing success, you train your mind to focus on positive outcomes and create a blueprint for your actions.

One of the key benefits of visualization is that it enhances your belief in yourself and your capabilities. When you consistently picture yourself succeeding, you strengthen your confidence and self-assurance. This positive mindset can help you overcome self-doubt, fears, and limiting beliefs that may hinder your progress.

Visualization also helps in clarifying your goals and aligning your actions with your desired outcomes. By mentally rehearsing the steps you need to take, you develop a clear roadmap for success. This process enables you to anticipate obstacles, devise strategies to overcome them, and make the necessary adjustments along the way.

Moreover, visualization activates the same neural pathways in your brain as actual experiences. When you vividly imagine yourself performing at your best, your brain sends signals to the corresponding muscles, creating a mind-body connection. This phenomenon enhances your physical and mental readiness, making it easier to execute your actions with precision and focus.

Visualization has been scientifically proven to enhance athletic performance and strength. Not only that but it has also been shown to reduce stress.

To incorporate visualization into your routine, find a quiet and comfortable space where you can relax. Close your eyes and engage your senses as you mentally create the scenario of achieving your goals. Visualize the sights, sounds, smells, and emotions associated with your success. Repeat this practice regularly, ideally before important events or during dedicated visualization sessions.

It's important to note that visualization alone isn't a magic solution. It serves as a complementary technique that amplifies your efforts and reinforces positive habits. Combine it with consistent action, proper planning, and effective strategies to maximize its impact on your success.

In conclusion, visualization and mental imagery can be transformative tools on your journey toward success. By harnessing the power of your mind to vividly imagine your desired outcomes, you enhance your confidence, clarify your goals, and align your actions. Make visualization a regular practice, and watch as it helps you unlock your full potential and achieve the success you desire.

Managing Negative Thoughts & Emotions

Negative thoughts and emotions are a natural part of life, but it's essential to develop strategies for managing them effectively. By learning how to navigate through negativity, you can cultivate resilience, maintain a positive mindset, and create a healthier emotional well-being. Here are some techniques to help you manage negative thoughts and emotions:

1. Mindfulness and Awareness: Practice being fully present in the moment and observing your thoughts and emotions without judgment. Mindfulness allows you to detach from negative thoughts and prevents them from overwhelming you. By increasing your awareness of your inner experiences, you can choose how to respond to them more consciously.

2. Reframing: Challenge negative thoughts and reframe them in a more positive or realistic light. Replace self-defeating or limiting beliefs with empowering and supportive ones. For example, instead of thinking, "I always fail," reframe it as, "I have the ability to learn and grow from my experiences."

3. Cognitive Restructuring: Identify and restructure negative thought patterns. This technique involves examining the evidence for and against your negative thoughts, considering alternative perspectives, and replacing irrational thoughts with more rational and balanced ones. This helps you gain a more realistic and positive outlook.

4. Emotional Expression: Find healthy ways to express and release negative emotions. Write in a journal, talk to a trusted friend, or engage in creative outlets such as art, music, or physical activities.

Expressing your emotions helps prevent them from bottling up and becoming overwhelming.

5. Self-Compassion: Treat yourself with kindness and understanding when negative thoughts or emotions arise. Practice self-compassion by acknowledging that everyone experiences difficulties and that it's okay to struggle. Offer yourself support and encouragement, just as you would for a close friend facing a similar situation.

6. Relaxation Techniques: Use relaxation techniques such as deep breathing exercises, progressive muscle relaxation, or meditation to calm your mind and body. These practices help reduce stress, alleviate anxiety, and promote a sense of inner peace.

7. Engaging in Positive Activities: Focus on activities that bring you joy, fulfillment, and a sense of accomplishment. Engaging in hobbies, exercise, spending time in nature, or connecting with loved ones can help shift your focus away from negative thoughts and emotions.

Managing negative thoughts and emotions is an ongoing practice. Be patient with yourself as you develop these techniques and implement them into your daily life. With time and consistency, you can cultivate a more positive and resilient mindset, allowing you to navigate challenges with greater ease and maintain both your physical and emotional health.

X: Supplements
Creatine

Creatine is a naturally occurring compound found in small amounts in various foods, particularly meat and fish. It plays a crucial role in the production of adenosine triphosphate (ATP), which is the primary source of energy for muscle contractions during intense exercise. One of the most well-researched and effective supplements for muscle building, creatine has been shown to provide several benefits:

1. Increased Muscle Strength and Power: Creatine supplementation has consistently demonstrated improvements in strength and power output, making it a popular choice among athletes and bodybuilders. It allows you to lift heavier weights, perform more repetitions, and generate greater muscular force.

2. Enhanced Exercise Performance: By increasing the availability of ATP, creatine helps to replenish energy stores more rapidly during high-intensity activities. This can lead to improved performance in short-duration, explosive exercises like weightlifting, sprinting, and jumping.

3. Increased Muscle Size: Creatine promotes muscle hydration by drawing water into the muscle cells, resulting in a fuller and more volumized appearance. This increase in intracellular fluid may contribute to muscle growth and a more pronounced muscular physique.

4. Faster Muscle Recovery: Creatine has been found to reduce muscle damage and inflammation, allowing for faster recovery between workouts. This can help you train more frequently and

consistently, leading to greater gains in muscle mass and strength over time.

5. Neuroprotective Benefits: Beyond its effects on muscle performance, creatine has shown potential neuroprotective properties. It may help protect and support brain health, enhance cognitive function, and provide benefits for conditions such as Parkinson's disease and depression. However, more research is needed to fully understand these effects.

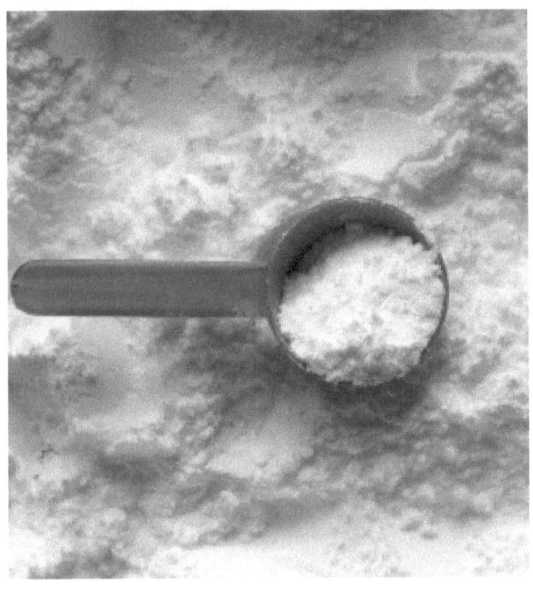

When supplementing with creatine, it is typically recommended to consume 3-5 grams per day. Some people prefer to undergo a loading phase to see faster results. During the loading phase, a higher dosage of creatine is consumed (usually around 20 grams per day) for a week to saturate the muscles with creatine. This is then followed by a maintenance phase, where a lower dosage (typically 3-5 grams per day) is taken to maintain elevated creatine levels in the muscles. With or without a loading phase, you'll still achieve the same result.

With a dose of 5g per day, it can take approximately 30 days to achieve full saturation. With a loading phase, it takes 5-7 days to achieve the same, full saturation. After that, follow up with a maintenance phase as said earlier.

Creatine monohydrate is the most common and widely studied form of creatine, and it is generally regarded as safe for most individuals when used as directed. However, it's important to note that individual responses to creatine may vary, and it may not be suitable for everyone. Consulting with a healthcare professional or registered dietitian is advisable before starting any new supplementation regimen.

To maximize the benefits of creatine supplementation, it is recommended to combine it with a well-balanced diet and a consistent resistance training program. Adequate hydration is also important when using creatine, as it may cause slight water retention. Overall, creatine is a widely recognized and effective supplement for enhancing strength, power, and muscle growth, and it is commonly used by athletes and individuals looking to improve their physical performance.

Protein

Protein is an essential macronutrient that plays a crucial role in building, repairing, and maintaining tissues in the body, including muscles, bones, and skin. While it's best to obtain protein from whole food sources such as lean meats, poultry, fish, dairy products, legumes, and nuts, protein supplements can be a convenient and effective way to meet your protein needs, especially for individuals with increased protein requirements or limited dietary options.

Here are some key points about protein supplementation:

1. Muscle Building and Recovery: Protein is often associated with muscle building and recovery due to its role in supporting muscle protein synthesis. Adequate protein intake, in combination with resistance training, is important for optimizing muscle growth, strength, and recovery. Protein supplements provide a convenient source of high-quality protein, which can be beneficial for individuals looking to enhance their muscle-building efforts.

2. Protein Quality and Types: Protein supplements come in various forms, such as whey protein, casein protein, soy protein, pea protein, and others. Whey protein is one of the most popular and widely available forms and is derived from milk. It is quickly absorbed by the body and rich in essential amino acids, making it an excellent choice for post-workout recovery. Casein protein, on the other hand, is digested more slowly, providing a sustained release of amino acids to support muscle repair and growth over an extended period.

3. Convenience and Portability: Protein supplements offer a convenient and portable option to increase protein intake, especially for those with busy lifestyles or limited time for meal preparation. They can be easily mixed with water or other beverages and

consumed on the go, making them a practical choice for individuals who need a quick and convenient protein source.

4. Protein Requirements and Timing: The recommended protein intake varies depending on factors such as age, sex, activity level, and goals. While protein needs can typically be met through a well-balanced diet, supplementation can be beneficial for those who struggle to consume adequate protein through food alone or have increased protein requirements. It's important to spread protein intake evenly throughout the day and include a source of protein in each meal to support muscle protein synthesis and maintain a positive nitrogen balance.

5. Safety and Considerations: Protein supplements are generally safe for healthy individuals when used as directed. However, it's essential to choose reputable brands and be mindful of the ingredients, as some supplements may contain added sugars, artificial flavors, or unnecessary additives. If you have any specific dietary restrictions or underlying health conditions, it's recommended to consult with a healthcare professional or registered dietitian before incorporating protein supplements into your routine.

While protein supplementation can be beneficial, it's important to remember that it should supplement a well-balanced diet and not replace whole food sources of protein. Whole foods provide additional essential nutrients, fiber, and other bioactive compounds that are important for overall health and well-being. Therefore, it's advisable to prioritize whole food sources of protein whenever possible and use protein supplements as a convenient option to meet specific dietary needs or goals.

Mass Gainers

Mass gainer powders are a type of dietary supplement designed to help individuals increase their calorie and protein intake to support muscle mass and weight gain. Here are some key points and pros of mass gainer powders:

1. Calorie and Macronutrient Dense: Mass gainer powders are formulated to be calorie-dense, providing a higher amount of calories per serving compared to regular protein powders. They typically contain a mix of carbohydrates, proteins, and fats to provide a substantial calorie boost. This makes them suitable for individuals who struggle to consume enough calories from their regular diet alone to support weight gain or muscle growth.

2. Protein Content: Mass gainer powders often contain a significant amount of protein, which is crucial for muscle repair and growth. The protein source may vary depending on the brand and product, commonly including whey protein, casein protein, or a blend of different protein sources. The protein content in mass gainers can range from 20 to 50 grams per serving or even higher.

3. Carbohydrate Source: Carbohydrates are an essential component of mass gainer powders as they provide the necessary energy to fuel workouts and support weight gain. These carbohydrates typically come from sources like maltodextrin, dextrose, or other fast-digesting carbohydrates to promote quick energy replenishment and muscle glycogen replenishment after intense exercise.

4. Healthy Fats: Some mass gainer powders may include healthy fats, such as MCT oil or omega-3 fatty acids, to contribute to the overall calorie content and provide additional nutritional benefits. These

fats help with nutrient absorption, hormone production, and overall health.

5. Additional Ingredients: Mass gainer powders may also contain additional ingredients such as vitamins, minerals, creatine, and other performance-enhancing compounds. These ingredients aim to support muscle recovery, energy production, and overall well-being.

6. Serving Size and Timing: The recommended serving size of mass gainer powders can vary depending on individual needs and goals. It's important to follow the instructions provided by the manufacturer to determine the appropriate serving size. Mass gainer powders are commonly consumed as a post-workout shake or between meals to provide an additional calorie and nutrient boost.

7. Considerations and Usage: While mass gainer powders can be beneficial for individuals who struggle to meet their calorie and protein needs, it's important to consider individual dietary requirements and goals. It's advisable to choose a mass gainer powder from a reputable brand, ensure it fits your specific nutritional needs, and consult with a healthcare professional or registered dietitian if you have any underlying health conditions or concerns.

While mass gainer powders can be beneficial for those looking to increase calorie and protein intake, it's important to consider some potential drawbacks and limitations. Here are some cons associated with mass gainers:

1. High-Calorie Content: Mass gainer powders are specifically designed to be calorie-dense, which can be a disadvantage for individuals who don't require a significant increase in calories. Consuming excessive calories beyond your needs can lead to unwanted weight gain, including fat mass. It's crucial to determine your calorie requirements and adjust your intake accordingly.

2. Processed Carbohydrates: Many mass gainer powders rely on processed carbohydrates as a source of calories. These carbohydrates are often refined and can include ingredients like maltodextrin, dextrose, or other sugars. While they provide quick energy, they lack the nutritional benefits found in whole food sources of carbohydrates, such as fiber and micronutrients.

3. Artificial Ingredients: Some mass gainer powders may contain artificial flavors, sweeteners, and additives to enhance taste and texture. These artificial ingredients may not align with everyone's preference for natural and whole food-based products. Additionally, certain individuals may be sensitive or allergic to specific artificial additives, which can cause digestive discomfort or other adverse reactions.

4. Digestive Issues: Due to the high calorie and macronutrient content, some individuals may experience digestive issues when consuming mass gainer powders. The concentrated nature of the powders, particularly if consumed in large quantities, can lead to bloating, gas, or an upset stomach. It's essential to start with smaller servings and gradually increase as tolerated.

5. Individual Tolerance and Sensitivity: Everyone's body responds differently to supplements, including mass gainers. Some individuals may find it challenging to tolerate the concentrated amounts of protein or carbohydrates found in these products. It's important to listen to your body and assess any potential negative reactions or discomfort.

6. Not a Substitute for Whole Foods: While mass gainer powders can provide a convenient way to increase calorie and protein intake, they should not replace a balanced and varied diet consisting of whole food sources. Whole foods offer a wide range of essential

nutrients, fiber, and phytochemicals that are beneficial for muscle gain and overall health.

It's crucial to weigh the pros and cons of mass gainer powders and consider your individual needs, goals, and preferences. If you're considering incorporating a mass gainer into your routine, it's advisable to choose a product from a reputable brand, read the ingredient label carefully, and opt for options with fewer artificial ingredients and processed carbohydrates.

Remember, the best approach is always to prioritize a well-rounded diet consisting of whole, nutrient-dense foods. Mass gainer powders should be viewed as a supplement to support your nutritional needs when necessary, and it's essential to consult with a healthcare professional or registered dietitian before making any significant changes to your diet or supplementation routine.

Mass gainer powders should not be viewed as a magic solution for muscle gain or weight gain. They should be used in conjunction with a well-rounded diet and a structured training program tailored to your goals. Whole food sources should still form the foundation of your nutrition plan, and mass gainer powders can be used as a convenient supplement to support your calorie and protein intake when needed.

If you want a convenient way to get extra calories and macros in, you'd be better off buying a high-quality protein powder and making mass gainer shakes with some added natural ingredients by yourself.

Here's a simple recipe for a homemade mass gainer shake that you can easily prepare:

Ingredients:

- 1 cup of milk (dairy or plant-based)

- 1 scoop of protein powder (flavor of your choice)

- 2 tablespoons of natural peanut butter

- 1/4 cup of rolled oats

- 1 ripe banana (optional)

- 1 tablespoon of honey or maple syrup (optional)

- Ice cubes (optional, for a chilled shake)

Instructions:

1. Add the milk to a blender or shaker bottle.

2. Add the protein powder, natural peanut butter, rolled oats, and ripe banana (if using) to the blender.

3. Optionally, you can add a tablespoon of honey or maple syrup for added taste and calories.

4. Blend all the ingredients until you achieve a smooth and creamy consistency. If using a shaker bottle, close the lid tightly and shake vigorously until well combined.

5. If desired, you can add a few ice cubes to the blender to make the shake colder and more refreshing.

6. Pour the mass gainer shake into a glass and enjoy!

This homemade mass gainer shake provides a balanced combination of protein, healthy fats from peanut butter, complex carbohydrates from oats, and essential nutrients. Adjust the quantities of ingredients based on your calorie and macronutrient needs. You can also customize the recipe by adding other ingredients such as Greek yogurt, flaxseeds, or berries for additional flavor and nutrition.

Remember to consider your overall dietary needs and consult with a healthcare professional or registered dietitian if you have specific nutritional requirements or allergies.

BCAAs and Amino Acid Blends

Branch Chain Amino Acids, commonly known as BCAAs, have gained popularity in the fitness and bodybuilding community. They consist of three essential amino acids: leucine, isoleucine, and valine. These amino acids play a crucial role in muscle protein synthesis and are believed to promote muscle growth and enhance exercise performance. However, the effectiveness and necessity of BCAA supplementation have been a subject of debate among experts.

While BCAAs are indeed important for muscle protein synthesis, it's important to note that they are already present in most high-quality protein sources, such as meat, dairy, eggs, and plant-based protein sources like legumes. If you consume an adequate amount of protein in your diet, you are likely already getting enough BCAAs without the need for supplementation.

One of the main reasons BCAA supplements are often considered a waste of money is that they lack the complete spectrum of essential amino acids. Consuming only BCAAs neglects other important amino acids that are necessary for overall muscle growth, recovery, and various metabolic functions. It's important to prioritize a well-rounded protein intake that includes all essential amino acids, rather than focusing solely on BCAAs.

Furthermore, studies have shown that the timing and composition of protein intake are more critical factors for optimizing muscle protein synthesis than BCAA supplementation alone. Consuming a balanced meal or protein shake that contains a complete amino acid profile shortly after your workout can provide all the necessary building blocks for muscle repair and growth.

In conclusion, while BCAAs have their merits in specific situations, for most individuals who consume a well-balanced diet with sufficient protein intake, BCAA supplementation is unnecessary. Instead, focus on consuming quality protein sources that provide a complete amino acid profile, as this will cover your body's needs for muscle building and recovery. As always, it's best to consult with a healthcare professional or registered dietitian before starting any new supplementation regimen.

Pre-Workout

Pre-workout supplements are popular among individuals seeking an extra boost of energy, focus, and performance during their workouts. However, it's essential to be informed and cautious when choosing pre-workout products, as some may contain ingredients that can have negative effects or pose potential health risks. Here are some guidelines on how to evaluate and select pre-workout supplements wisely:

1. Research and read labels: Before purchasing a pre-workout supplement, conduct thorough research on the product and its ingredients. Look for reputable brands that provide detailed information about their formulations, including the specific ingredients and their quantities. Read the labels carefully to ensure transparency and understand what you are putting into your body.

2. Assess the ingredient profile: Pay attention to the ingredients in the pre-workout supplement. Look for evidence-based and well-studied ingredients that are safe and effective for enhancing exercise performance, such as caffeine, tyrosine, or citrulline. These ingredients can provide benefits like increased energy, improved endurance, and enhanced focus.

3. Avoid proprietary blends: Be cautious of pre-workout supplements that use proprietary blends, which group several ingredients without specifying their individual dosages. This lack of transparency makes it difficult to assess the effectiveness and safety of the product. Opt for supplements that provide clear information about the dosage of each ingredient.

4. Check for banned substances: Ensure that the pre-workout supplement is tested by a reputable third-party organization for the

presence of banned substances. Look for certifications such as Informed-Sport or NSF Certified for Sport, which verify the product's quality and absence of prohibited substances.

5. Assess tolerance and sensitivity: Understand your individual tolerance and sensitivity to stimulants like caffeine. Some pre-workout supplements contain high amounts of caffeine, which can have different effects on individuals. If you are sensitive to stimulants or have certain health conditions, choose a pre-workout with a lower caffeine content or opt for stimulant-free alternatives.

6. Consider your goals: Select a pre-workout supplement that aligns with your specific fitness goals. Different products may have different formulations targeting specific outcomes, such as energy and endurance, muscle pump, or focus and cognition. Determine which benefits are most important to you and choose a product accordingly.

7. Consult a healthcare professional: If you have any underlying health conditions, are taking medications, or have concerns about using pre-workout supplements, it's advisable to consult with a healthcare professional before incorporating them into your routine. They can provide personalized guidance and ensure compatibility with your circumstances.

Remember, while pre-workout supplements can provide temporary benefits, they should not be relied upon as a substitute for a well-balanced diet and proper training program. Prioritize overall nutrition, sleep, hydration, and consistency in your training routine for long-term progress and optimal performance.

Fat Burners

I am not particularly against all fat burners, as long as people understand the context. If you have a proper and consistent diet and training routine, you're in a caloric deficit, and if you then add in a few extra compounds to slightly enhance your calorie expenditure and suppress appetite by a little then that's fine. You might end up with a minor fat-loss increase. But relying on it and thinking it will magically make you lose fat by itself is not smart. If you have the extra money, already do all the necessary things, and want to completely maximize things, go for it if you'd like. But for the average person, it's a completely unnecessary supplement and you should rather focus on getting the big things right.

Here are some reasons why fat burners are often considered a waste of money:

1. Limited evidence of effectiveness: The effectiveness of fat burners in promoting significant and sustainable weight loss is questionable. Many fat burners rely on a combination of stimulants, herbal extracts, and other ingredients to potentially increase metabolism, suppress appetite, or enhance fat oxidation. However, scientific evidence supporting their efficacy is often limited, inconsistent, or based on short-term studies.

2. Minimal impact on overall weight loss: Even if fat burners have some modest effects on metabolism or fat oxidation, their impact on overall weight loss is usually minimal. Weight loss primarily depends on achieving a calorie deficit through a combination of proper nutrition and regular physical activity. Relying solely on fat burners without addressing the underlying factors contributing to weight gain or lack of progress is unlikely to yield significant results.

3. Potential health risks: Fat burners often contain stimulants, such as caffeine, ephedrine, or synephrine, which can increase heart rate, blood pressure, and have other adverse effects. Moreover, the long-term safety of some ingredients in fat burners remains uncertain, as they may not undergo rigorous testing or regulation. Individuals with underlying health conditions or sensitivities to stimulants should exercise caution and consult a healthcare professional before using such supplements.

4. Focus on short-term fixes: Fat burners tend to promote the idea of quick fixes and instant results. However, sustainable weight loss and overall health improvements require a holistic approach that includes balanced nutrition, regular physical activity, adequate sleep, stress management, and lifestyle modifications. Relying solely on fat burners may divert attention from addressing these fundamental aspects and create an unsustainable mindset.

5. Potential for dependency and tolerance: Some fat burners contain stimulants that can lead to dependency and tolerance over time. This means that the initial effects of increased energy, focus, and appetite suppression may diminish as the body becomes accustomed to the ingredients. Consequently, individuals may need to increase the dosage or seek stronger formulations, which can further compromise their health and well-being.

6. Cost and financial investment: Fat burners can be expensive, especially when considering long-term use. Spending money on these supplements without obtaining significant and sustainable results can lead to frustration and a waste of financial resources. Allocating those funds toward nutritious food, training equipment, or other supportive services will yield greater benefits for overall health and weight management.

Instead of relying on fat burners, focus on adopting healthy lifestyle habits that support sustainable weight loss and overall well-being. Prioritize a balanced diet rich in whole foods, regular physical activity, adequate sleep, stress management techniques, and mindful eating. Consult with a healthcare professional or registered dietitian for personalized guidance on achieving your weight loss goals safely and sustainably. Remember, there are no magic pills for weight loss, and long-term success requires commitment, patience, and a comprehensive approach.

Testosterone-Boosters

Testosterone boosters are dietary supplements that claim to increase the production or availability of testosterone in the body. While there are natural compounds that have been shown to have some influence on testosterone levels, it's important to understand that the effects of testosterone boosters are often limited and may not lead to significant increases in muscle mass. Here are some points to consider:

1. Modest effects on testosterone levels: Testosterone boosters typically contain ingredients like herbal extracts, vitamins, and minerals that have shown some potential to influence testosterone production or activity. However, the observed effects are often modest and temporary. Studies have shown that the increase in testosterone levels associated with these supplements is generally small and may not translate into substantial gains in muscle mass or strength.

2. Individual variations: The response to testosterone boosters can vary significantly among individuals. Some people may experience a slight increase in testosterone levels, while others may not see any noticeable changes. Factors such as age, genetics, baseline testosterone levels, overall health, and lifestyle habits can influence the response to these supplements.

3. Lack of evidence for muscle mass gains: Despite the claims made by manufacturers, the scientific evidence supporting the use of testosterone boosters for significant muscle mass gains is limited. While higher testosterone levels can support muscle growth, testosterone boosters do not produce results significant enough to get any noticeable benefits in muscle growth or fat loss. It's important to note that testosterone is just one of many factors

involved in muscle development. Proper nutrition, adequate protein intake, progressive resistance training, and overall calorie balance play more significant roles in building muscle mass.

4. Potential side effects: Testosterone boosters, especially those containing synthetic ingredients, can carry potential risks and side effects. These may include hormonal imbalances, liver toxicity, cardiovascular complications, acne, mood swings, and disruptions in natural hormone production. It's crucial to consult with a healthcare professional before considering the use of testosterone boosters, especially if you have any underlying health conditions or are taking other medications.

5. Natural methods for optimizing testosterone levels: Instead of relying solely on testosterone boosters, there are several natural methods you can incorporate to support optimal testosterone levels. These include maintaining a balanced and nutritious diet, engaging in regular physical activity and strength training, managing stress levels, getting enough quality sleep, maintaining a healthy weight, and avoiding excessive alcohol consumption and smoking. These lifestyle factors can have a more significant and sustainable impact on testosterone levels and overall health.

It's important to approach testosterone boosters with realistic expectations. While they may have a minor influence on testosterone levels, their effects on muscle mass gains are likely to be minimal. If you have concerns about low testosterone levels or desire significant muscle growth, it's recommended to consult with a healthcare professional who can provide appropriate guidance and explore other strategies that may be more effective and safe for achieving your goals.

Fish Oil

Fish oil supplementation has gained popularity due to its potential health benefits, particularly its rich content of omega-3 fatty acids. Here are some key points to consider about fish oil supplementation:

1. Omega-3 fatty acids: Fish oil is a rich source of omega-3 fatty acids, including eicosapentaenoic acid (EPA) and docosahexaenoic acid (DHA). These fatty acids play crucial roles in supporting overall health, including brain function, heart health, and reducing inflammation in the body.

2. Heart health benefits: Omega-3 fatty acids have been extensively studied for their positive impact on cardiovascular health. They have been shown to lower triglyceride levels, reduce blood pressure, decrease the risk of heart disease, and improve overall heart function.

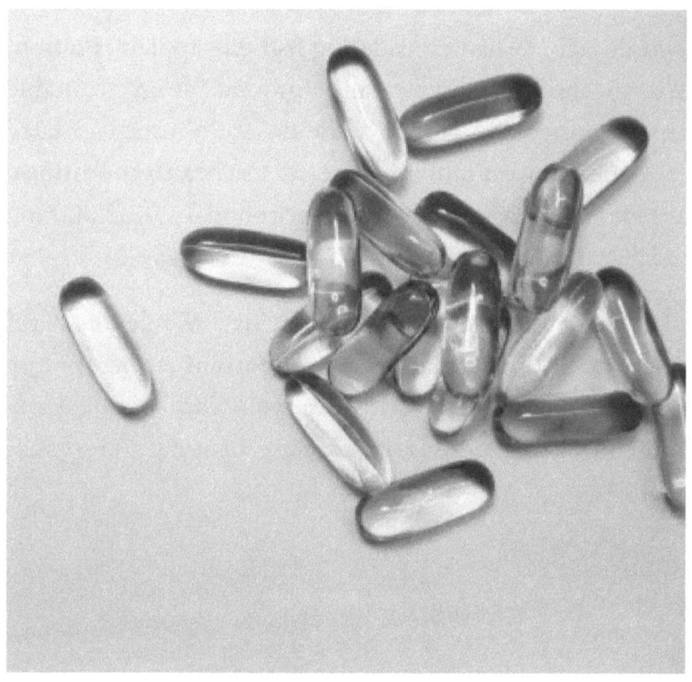

3. Anti-inflammatory properties: Omega-3 fatty acids have potent anti-inflammatory effects on the body. They can help reduce inflammation, which is a common underlying factor in various chronic conditions such as arthritis, inflammatory bowel disease, and even certain types of cancer.

4. Brain health and cognitive function: DHA, one of the omega-3 fatty acids found in fish oil, is a major structural component of the brain. Adequate intake of DHA has been associated with improved cognitive function, memory, and overall brain health. It may also play a role in reducing the risk of age-related cognitive decline and neurodegenerative diseases.

5. Joint health and exercise recovery: Fish oil supplementation has shown promise in supporting joint health and reducing symptoms of joint stiffness and discomfort. It may also aid in exercise recovery by reducing inflammation and promoting muscle repair.

6. Quality and dosage: When considering fish oil supplementation, it's important to choose a high-quality product from reputable sources to ensure purity and potency. The dosage of omega-3 fatty acids can vary depending on individual needs and health conditions, but a typical recommendation is to aim for around 1,000-2,000 mg of combined EPA and DHA per day.

7. Dietary sources of omega-3 fatty acids: While fish oil supplementation can be beneficial, it's also important to incorporate dietary sources of omega-3 fatty acids into your eating plan. Fatty fish like salmon, mackerel, and sardines are excellent natural sources of EPA and DHA.

Vitamin D

Vitamin D is a fat-soluble vitamin that plays a crucial role in various physiological functions within the body. It is primarily known for its role in supporting bone health and promoting the absorption of calcium and phosphorus. However, emerging research suggests that vitamin D has far-reaching effects beyond skeletal health.

One of the primary sources of vitamin D is sunlight. When our skin is exposed to sunlight, it triggers the synthesis of vitamin D3, also known as cholecalciferol. Additionally, vitamin D can be obtained through certain foods such as fatty fish (e.g., salmon, mackerel), fortified dairy products, eggs, and mushrooms.

Here are some key points about vitamin D and its potential benefits:

1. Bone health: Vitamin D plays a crucial role in calcium metabolism and bone mineralization. It aids in the absorption of calcium and phosphorus from the intestine, helps regulate their levels in the blood, and promotes the deposition of these minerals into bones, thus contributing to overall bone strength.

2. Immune function: Vitamin D is involved in modulating the immune system and has been linked to a reduced risk of autoimmune diseases, such as multiple sclerosis and rheumatoid arthritis. Adequate vitamin D levels may also support immune responses against infections.

3. Muscle function: Vitamin D is important for muscle health and function. It plays a role in muscle protein synthesis, muscle strength, and coordination. Low levels of vitamin D have been associated with an increased risk of muscle weakness, falls, and fractures, particularly in older adults.

4. Mood and mental health: Some studies have suggested a link between vitamin D deficiency and an increased risk of mood disorders, such as depression and seasonal affective disorder (SAD). While the exact mechanisms are not fully understood, it is thought that vitamin D may influence neurotransmitter function and have a positive impact on mental well-being.

5. Heart health: Research has shown a potential connection between vitamin D deficiency and an increased risk of cardiovascular diseases, including hypertension, heart disease, and stroke. Adequate vitamin D levels may help maintain healthy blood pressure and reduce the risk of these conditions.

6. Cancer prevention: Although more research is needed, some studies have suggested that vitamin D may play a role in cancer prevention. It may help regulate cell growth, promote apoptosis (cell death) of cancer cells, and inhibit the development of blood vessels that support tumor growth.

It is important to note that vitamin D deficiency is common, especially in regions with limited sunlight exposure, during winter months, or among individuals with limited dietary intake. Additionally, certain factors such as age, skin pigmentation, and obesity can affect vitamin D synthesis and absorption.

If you suspect a deficiency or are considering vitamin D supplementation, it is advisable to consult with a healthcare professional. They can assess your individual needs, recommend appropriate supplementation, and monitor your vitamin D levels over time. Remember that maintaining optimal vitamin D levels should be part of a comprehensive approach to overall health, including a balanced diet, regular sun exposure, and a healthy lifestyle.

Magnesium

Magnesium is an essential mineral that plays a vital role in numerous physiological processes within the body. It is involved in over 300 enzymatic reactions and is necessary for proper muscle and nerve function, energy production, protein synthesis, and maintenance of healthy bones and teeth.

While magnesium can be obtained from various food sources such as green leafy vegetables, nuts, seeds, and whole grains, many people may still have inadequate magnesium intake due to factors such as poor diet, certain medical conditions, or medications that can affect magnesium absorption.

Supplementing with magnesium can be beneficial for several reasons:

1. Muscle and nerve function: Magnesium is necessary for proper muscle contraction and relaxation. It helps regulate the electrical impulses that allow muscles to contract and contributes to the normal functioning of the nervous system. Adequate magnesium levels may help reduce muscle cramps, spasms, and restless leg syndrome.

2. Energy production: Magnesium is involved in the production and utilization of ATP (adenosine triphosphate), which is the primary source of energy in cells. It is a cofactor for several enzymes involved in energy metabolism, making it essential for energy production and maintenance of optimal cellular function.

3. Bone health: Magnesium works in conjunction with calcium and vitamin D to promote healthy bone development and maintenance. It aids in the absorption and metabolism of calcium and helps regulate calcium levels in the body. Adequate magnesium levels

contribute to strong bones and may help reduce the risk of osteoporosis.

4. Heart health: Magnesium plays a crucial role in maintaining a healthy cardiovascular system. It helps regulate heart rhythm, supports blood vessel function, and assists in blood pressure regulation. Some research suggests that magnesium supplementation may help lower blood pressure and reduce the risk of cardiovascular diseases.

5. Relaxation and stress management: Magnesium has calming properties and is often referred to as a natural relaxant. It plays a role in the regulation of neurotransmitters and helps balance the stress response. Adequate magnesium levels may contribute to better sleep quality, relaxation, and overall stress management.

When considering magnesium supplementation, it is important to choose the appropriate form of magnesium. There are various types of magnesium supplements available, including magnesium citrate, magnesium oxide, magnesium glycinate, and more. Each form has different absorption rates and bioavailability, so it is advisable to consult with a healthcare professional to determine the most suitable option for your needs.

It is also important to note that excessive magnesium supplementation can lead to gastrointestinal discomfort or other side effects. Therefore, it is recommended to follow the recommended dosage guidelines and consult with a healthcare professional before starting any new supplementation regimen, particularly if you have any underlying health conditions or are taking medications.

In conclusion, magnesium supplementation can be beneficial for individuals who have inadequate magnesium intake or specific health concerns. It supports various physiological functions, including muscle and nerve function, energy production, bone health, heart health, and stress management. Choosing the right form of magnesium and consulting with a healthcare professional are essential for safe and effective supplementation.

Vitamin C

Vitamin C, also known as ascorbic acid, is a water-soluble vitamin that plays a crucial role in maintaining overall health and well-being. It is a powerful antioxidant that helps protect the body against damage from harmful free radicals and supports various physiological functions.

Here are some key benefits and functions of vitamin C:

1. Immune system support: Vitamin C is well-known for its immune-boosting properties. It plays a vital role in the production and function of white blood cells, which are essential for a healthy immune response. Adequate vitamin C levels can help strengthen the immune system and protect against common infections and illnesses.

2. Antioxidant protection: As an antioxidant, vitamin C helps neutralize free radicals, which are unstable molecules that can cause oxidative stress and damage to cells. By scavenging these free radicals, vitamin C helps protect against chronic diseases such as heart disease, certain cancers, and age-related degenerative conditions.

3. Collagen synthesis: Vitamin C is essential for the synthesis of collagen, a protein that provides structure and strength to various tissues in the body, including the skin, bones, tendons, and blood vessels. Adequate vitamin C levels support healthy skin, wound healing, and the maintenance of strong and flexible connective tissues.

4. Iron absorption: Vitamin C enhances the absorption of nonheme iron, which is the type of iron found in plant-based foods and iron supplements. It helps convert iron into a form that is more easily

absorbed by the body, improving iron status and preventing iron deficiency anemia.

5. Antioxidant regeneration: Vitamin C helps regenerate other antioxidants in the body, such as vitamin E. By replenishing these antioxidants, vitamin C ensures their continuous antioxidant activity, providing ongoing protection against oxidative damage.

6. Brain health: Vitamin C is involved in the synthesis of neurotransmitters, such as dopamine and norepinephrine, which are important for mood regulation and cognitive function. Adequate vitamin C levels may contribute to better brain health, mental well-being, and a reduced risk of age-related cognitive decline.

It is important to note that vitamin C is not produced or stored in the body, so it must be obtained from dietary sources or supplements regularly. Good food sources of vitamin C include citrus fruits, berries, kiwi, bell peppers, broccoli, and leafy green vegetables.

While vitamin C supplementation is generally safe, it is recommended to meet your daily vitamin C needs through a balanced diet whenever possible. However, certain individuals may benefit from vitamin C supplements, such as those with limited dietary intake, malabsorption issues, or specific health conditions. It is always advisable to consult with a healthcare professional before starting any new supplementation regimen.

Prebiotics and Probiotics

Probiotics and prebiotics play important roles in promoting a healthy gut and overall well-being. They are commonly referred to as "good bacteria" and "food for the good bacteria," respectively. Let's explore what probiotics and prebiotics are and how their supplementation can benefit your health.

Probiotics are live microorganisms that, when consumed in adequate amounts, confer health benefits on the host. They include strains of beneficial bacteria like Lactobacillus and Bifidobacterium, which naturally occur in the gut and help maintain a balanced microbial ecosystem. Probiotics can also be found in fermented foods like yogurt, sauerkraut, and kimchi.

The benefits of probiotics include:

1. Improved gut health: Probiotics help restore and maintain a healthy balance of beneficial bacteria in the gut, which is essential for proper digestion, nutrient absorption, and overall gut health. They can help alleviate symptoms of digestive issues such as bloating, gas, and diarrhea.

2. Enhanced immune function: A significant portion of the immune system resides in the gut. Probiotics support the immune system by promoting the growth of beneficial bacteria, which can help reduce the risk of certain infections and enhance immune response.

3. Relief from antibiotic-associated side effects: Antibiotics can disrupt the natural balance of gut bacteria, leading to digestive issues and increased susceptibility to infections. Taking probiotics during or after a course of antibiotics can help restore the balance of gut bacteria and minimize the side effects.

Prebiotics, on the other hand, are non-digestible fibers that serve as food for the beneficial bacteria in the gut. They can be found in various plant-based foods, such as bananas, onions, garlic, asparagus, and whole grains. Prebiotics nourish the existing probiotic bacteria in the gut, allowing them to thrive and perform their beneficial functions.

The benefits of prebiotics include:

1. Gut health support: Prebiotics provide nourishment to the beneficial bacteria in the gut, promoting their growth and activity. This helps maintain a healthy gut environment and supports optimal digestion and nutrient absorption.

2. Increased probiotic effectiveness: Prebiotics act as a fuel source for probiotic bacteria, enhancing their survival and activity in the gut. When consumed together, probiotics and prebiotics create a symbiotic relationship, maximizing the benefits of both.

Supplementation with probiotics and prebiotics can be beneficial for individuals who may not consume enough of these components through their regular diet. Probiotic and prebiotic supplements are available in various forms, including capsules, powders, and fermented food products.

When considering probiotic and prebiotic supplementation, it's important to:

1. Choose a reputable brand: Look for supplements that contain specific strains of probiotic bacteria and have undergone quality testing to ensure viability and safety.

2. Select the right strains: Different probiotic strains have different functions and benefits. Choose a supplement with strains that are

known to address your specific health concerns or support your overall well-being.

3. Follow dosage instructions: Take the recommended dosage as indicated on the supplement packaging or as advised by a healthcare professional. Dosages may vary depending on the specific product and your health needs.

4. Incorporate a variety of prebiotic-rich foods: While prebiotic supplements are available, it's also important to include a diverse range of prebiotic-rich foods in your diet. This ensures you receive a wide spectrum of prebiotic fibers to support the growth of different beneficial bacteria.

As with any dietary supplement, it's advisable to consult with a healthcare professional before starting probiotic or prebiotic supplementation, especially if you have underlying health conditions or are taking other medications.

In conclusion, probiotics and prebiotics are valuable components for promoting a healthy gut and overall well-being. Probiotics help restore and maintain a balanced gut microbiome, while prebiotics provide nourishment to the beneficial bacteria. Supplementation can be beneficial for individuals who may have limited dietary intake or specific health concerns. By incorporating probiotic-rich foods, prebiotic-rich foods, and appropriate supplements when necessary, you can support a healthy gut environment and optimize your digestive health.

Multivitamins

Many people see multivitamins as an incredible thing, after all only good things can come from covering all your vitamin and mineral bases with one simple pill, right? When diving into deeper research, your opinion on multivitamins might change.

Although multivitamins supplements technically have many micronutrients you need combined into one pill, it's not as beneficial as you may believe.

When looking at research, it has been proven that multivitamins don't do much at all. There is not enough evidence to say that multivitamins either make you live longer, protect you from diseases, or support your health in any other way.

Micronutrients are certainly very important, our body needs them to function properly. But, the only time supplementation becomes effective is when faced with deficiencies. A lot of times, people think they have deficiencies when they don't.

There are some common deficiencies like vitamin K, vitamin D, Iron, zinc, and magnesium deficiencies. The problem is that a multivitamin supplement wouldn't give you enough of these anyway. When dealing with deficiencies, you'd be much better by supplementing specifically for them. E.g., if you lack vitamin D, supplement it directly.

Even with all this evidence for the lack of multivitamin benefits, they are still very popular due to their marketing. All they have to say is "Take this one pill and it will fill in all of your nutrition gaps" even though it won't, and it's hard to believe it won't because it technically has many of the micronutrients your body needs.

Focus on getting enough macronutrients from a balanced diet, also containing fruits and vegetables. Multivitamins can never outweigh a poor diet, no matter how much you take them.

How To Incorporate Supplements Into Your Nutrition Plan

Incorporating supplements into your nutrition plan can be an effective way to support your overall health and reach specific goals. Here are some strategies to consider when incorporating supplements into your nutrition plan:

1. Assess your needs: Start by assessing your individual needs and goals. Consider factors such as your age, sex, activity level, dietary restrictions, and any specific health concerns you may have. This will help you determine which supplements may be beneficial for you.

2. Seek professional advice: It's always a good idea to consult with a healthcare professional, such as a registered dietitian or doctor, before starting any new supplements. They can provide personalized recommendations based on your specific needs and ensure that the supplements you choose are safe and appropriate for you.

3. Prioritize whole foods: Remember that supplements should not replace a balanced diet rich in whole, nutrient-dense foods. Supplements are meant to complement a healthy diet, not serve as a substitute for it. Focus on consuming a variety of fruits, vegetables, lean proteins, whole grains, and healthy fats to meet your nutritional needs.

4. Choose quality products: When selecting supplements, opt for reputable brands that prioritize quality, safety, and transparency. Look for third-party certifications, such as NSF International or USP, to ensure that the products have been tested for purity and accuracy of ingredients. Read product labels and ingredient lists to understand what you're putting into your body.

5. Start with the basics: Begin with essential supplements that provide a solid foundation for overall health. These may include high-quality omega-3 fatty acids for heart and brain health, and vitamin D if you have limited sun exposure.

6. Consider specific needs: If you have specific dietary needs or health concerns, you may benefit from targeted supplements. For example, if you follow a plant-based diet, you might consider supplementing with vitamin B12, iron, or omega-3 fatty acids. If you have joint issues, glucosamine or collagen supplements may be helpful. Tailor your supplement choices to address your individual requirements.

7. Timing and dosage: Follow the recommended dosage instructions provided by the supplement manufacturer or as advised by your healthcare professional. Some supplements are best taken with meals, while others may be more effective on an empty stomach. Pay attention to timing guidelines to maximize their benefits.

8. Monitor and adjust: Keep track of your supplement intake and monitor how you feel and any changes in your health. If you're not experiencing the desired effects or are unsure about a particular supplement, consult with your healthcare professional for guidance. They can help you make adjustments as needed.

9. Be consistent: Consistency is key when it comes to supplements. Take them regularly and as directed to experience their potential benefits. Incorporate them into your daily routine to establish a consistent habit.

10. Periodic reevaluation: Regularly reassess your supplement regimen to ensure it aligns with your changing needs and goals. As your lifestyle, dietary habits, or health status evolve, you may need to adjust or discontinue certain supplements.

Remember, supplements are not magic solutions and should not replace a balanced diet or a healthy lifestyle. They should complement your overall nutrition plan and be used strategically to fill in nutrient gaps or address specific needs. Focus on a well-rounded approach that includes a nutrient-rich diet, regular physical activity, adequate sleep, and stress management for optimal health and well-being.

XI: Hormone Optimization

Hormones play a crucial role in your overall health and fitness, including muscle building and fat loss. Hormones like testosterone, estrogen, insulin, and cortisol can impact your energy levels, metabolism, mood, and body composition.

In this chapter, we'll explore the factors that can affect your hormone levels, including nutrition, exercise, stress, sleep, and environmental factors. We'll also discuss the different types of hormone imbalances and their potential effects on your health.

We'll then dive into strategies for optimizing your hormone levels naturally, including diet and lifestyle modifications, supplementation, and hormone replacement therapy (HRT). We'll also touch on the importance of consulting with a qualified healthcare professional before making any significant changes to your hormone levels.

Understanding Hormones

Hormones are chemical messengers produced by various glands and tissues in the body. They play a crucial role in regulating and coordinating numerous bodily functions, ensuring that different systems work together harmoniously. Hormones act as signaling molecules, traveling through the bloodstream to target specific cells or organs where they exert their effects.

The endocrine system, which includes glands such as the pituitary, thyroid, adrenal, and reproductive glands, is responsible for producing and releasing hormones. Each hormone has a specific function and target, and they work in concert to maintain balance and homeostasis within the body.

Hormones have a wide range of roles in the body, including:

1. Metabolism: Hormones influence metabolism by regulating energy production, storage, and utilization. For example, insulin regulates blood sugar levels and promotes the uptake and storage of glucose, while thyroid hormones regulate the overall metabolic rate.

2. Muscle Growth: Hormones such as testosterone, growth hormone, and insulin-like growth factor-1 (IGF-1) play vital roles in muscle growth and repair. They promote protein synthesis, enhance muscle cell signaling, and support the development of lean muscle mass.

3. Fat Loss: Hormones can influence fat metabolism and storage. For instance, hormones like adrenaline and noradrenaline increase fat mobilization, while insulin and cortisol can affect fat storage and distribution.

4. Energy Levels: Hormones impact energy levels by regulating the production and utilization of energy sources such as glucose and fatty acids. Hormonal imbalances can contribute to fatigue or fluctuations in energy levels.

5. Mood and Mental Health: Hormones can affect mood, emotions, and mental well-being. For example, serotonin, dopamine, and endorphins are neurotransmitters that play a role in regulating mood, while hormonal imbalances can contribute to mood swings, anxiety, or depression.

6. Libido and Sexual Function: Hormones, particularly sex hormones like testosterone, estrogen, and progesterone, influence sexual development, desire, and reproductive function. Imbalances in these hormones can impact libido and sexual health.

The precise effects of hormones vary depending on their type and target cells, and they often work in intricate feedback loops to maintain balance. Hormones are sensitive to internal and external factors, including stress, nutrition, sleep, exercise, and environmental cues.

Understanding the role of hormones in the body is essential for optimizing health and achieving fitness goals. By considering the influence of hormones on metabolism, muscle growth, fat loss, energy levels, mood, and libido, individuals can make informed choices about their lifestyle, nutrition, and training strategies to support hormone balance and overall well-being.

Key Hormones

Several hormones play significant roles in fitness, well-being, and overall health. Understanding the functions, sources, and effects of these hormones can help individuals optimize their body composition, strength, and performance. Here are some of the primary hormones relevant to fitness:

1. Testosterone: Testosterone is a key hormone for both men and women, primarily produced in the testes in men and ovaries in women. It supports muscle growth, strength, and bone density. Higher testosterone levels are associated with increased lean muscle mass, reduced body fat, and improved athletic performance.

2. Estrogen: Estrogen is the primary female sex hormone, mainly produced in the ovaries. It plays a crucial role in regulating the menstrual cycle and supporting reproductive health. Estrogen also influences bone density, metabolism, and body composition. In women, optimal estrogen levels are important for overall well-being and fitness.

3. Progesterone: Progesterone is another female sex hormone, primarily produced in the ovaries. It is essential for regulating the menstrual cycle, supporting pregnancy, and preparing the uterus for implantation. Progesterone also plays a role in metabolism and can affect water retention and mood.

4. Growth Hormone (GH): Growth hormone is produced by the pituitary gland and is involved in tissue growth, repair, and regeneration. It stimulates protein synthesis, promotes muscle growth, and helps maintain bone density. GH also aids in fat metabolism and can contribute to improved body composition.

5. Insulin: Insulin is produced by the pancreas and regulates blood sugar levels. It facilitates the uptake of glucose into cells, promotes energy storage, and supports muscle growth. Proper insulin function is vital for managing body weight, optimizing energy levels, and preventing metabolic disorders.

6. Cortisol: Cortisol, often referred to as the stress hormone, is produced by the adrenal glands. It helps the body respond to stress and regulates energy metabolism. However, chronically elevated cortisol levels can negatively impact muscle growth, increase fat storage, and hinder recovery.

7. Thyroid Hormones (T3 and T4): Thyroid hormones, produced by the thyroid gland, play a critical role in regulating metabolism. Triiodothyronine (T3) and thyroxine (T4) influence energy production, nutrient utilization, and body temperature. Imbalances in thyroid hormones can lead to changes in body weight, energy levels, and overall metabolic rate.

These hormones, along with others, work in synergy to regulate various physiological processes and influence body composition, strength, and performance.

Hormonal Imbalances

Hormonal imbalances can have a significant impact on overall health and fitness goals. Here are some common imbalances and their associated signs and symptoms:

1. Low Testosterone: Low testosterone levels, also known as hypogonadism, can affect both men and women. Symptoms may include reduced muscle mass, decreased strength, fatigue, low libido, mood changes, increased body fat, and decreased bone density. Low testosterone can hinder muscle growth, recovery, and overall performance.

2. Estrogen Dominance: Estrogen dominance occurs when there is an imbalance between estrogen and progesterone levels, often seen in women. Symptoms may include breast tenderness, irregular menstrual cycles, mood swings, weight gain, water retention, and decreased libido. Estrogen dominance can impact body composition and potentially lead to fat storage.

3. Thyroid Disorders: Thyroid disorders can manifest as hypothyroidism (underactive thyroid) or hyperthyroidism (overactive thyroid). Hypothyroidism may cause fatigue, weight gain, difficulty losing weight, dry skin, hair loss, and sluggish metabolism. Hyperthyroidism may lead to weight loss, increased heart rate, anxiety, insomnia, and heat intolerance. Thyroid disorders can influence energy levels, metabolic rate, and body composition.

4. Adrenal Dysfunction: Adrenal dysfunction, commonly known as adrenal fatigue or adrenal insufficiency, occurs when the adrenal glands struggle to produce adequate levels of cortisol. Symptoms may include chronic fatigue, difficulty managing stress, weakened immune function, sleep disturbances, and hormonal imbalances.

Adrenal dysfunction can impact energy levels, recovery, and overall well-being.

It's important to note that these imbalances can vary in severity and may require a medical assessment for an accurate diagnosis. If you suspect a hormonal imbalance, it's recommended to consult with a healthcare professional who specializes in hormone health. They can conduct appropriate tests, assess your symptoms, and provide tailored treatment options.

Addressing hormonal imbalances often involves a multifaceted approach, including lifestyle modifications, nutrition, stress management, and potential hormone replacement therapies under medical supervision. By addressing hormonal imbalances and restoring optimal hormone levels, individuals can enhance their overall health, improve fitness outcomes, and work towards achieving their goals more effectively.

Lifestyle Factors

Lifestyle factors play a crucial role in influencing hormone levels and balance. Here are some key factors to consider and strategies for optimizing them:

1. Nutrition: A balanced and nutrient-rich diet is essential for supporting healthy hormone levels. Include a variety of whole foods, including lean proteins, healthy fats, complex carbohydrates, and plenty of fruits and vegetables. Focus on foods that support hormonal health, such as those rich in omega-3 fatty acids, vitamins, and minerals. Minimize processed foods, refined sugars, and unhealthy fats, as they can negatively impact hormone balance.

2. Sleep: Quality sleep is vital for hormone regulation and overall well-being. Aim for 7-9 hours of uninterrupted sleep each night. Establish a consistent sleep schedule, create a relaxing bedtime routine, and ensure your sleep environment is conducive to restful sleep. Prioritize sleep hygiene practices, such as avoiding screens before bed, maintaining a cool and dark bedroom, and practicing relaxation techniques if needed.

3. Stress Management: Chronic stress can disrupt hormone balance. Implement stress management techniques such as meditation, deep breathing exercises, yoga, or engaging in hobbies that promote relaxation. Find healthy outlets for stress, such as regular physical activity, spending time in nature, or journaling. Prioritize self-care activities to reduce stress and promote overall well-being.

4. Exercise: Regular physical activity is beneficial for hormone regulation. Both aerobic exercise and strength training can positively impact hormone levels. Aim for a combination of cardiovascular workouts and resistance training to support overall fitness and

hormone balance. However, avoid excessive exercise or overtraining, as it can lead to hormonal imbalances. Find a balance that suits your individual needs and goals.

5. Environmental Factors: Be mindful of environmental factors that can disrupt hormone balance. Minimize exposure to endocrine-disrupting chemicals found in certain plastics, household products, and personal care items. Choose natural and non-toxic alternatives whenever possible. Be aware of potential hormone disruptors in your environment and take steps to reduce exposure.

Remember, hormone balance is a complex interplay of various factors, and it may take time to achieve optimal levels. It's important to listen to your body, make gradual changes, and seek guidance from healthcare professionals if needed. By adopting a holistic approach to lifestyle factors, you can support healthy hormone levels and enhance overall well-being.

Nutrition and Hormones

Nutrition plays a significant role in hormone production and regulation. Here are the key aspects to consider:

1. Macronutrient Balance: Consuming a balanced ratio of macronutrients, including carbohydrates, proteins, and fats, is crucial for hormone health. Each macronutrient plays a specific role in hormone production. For example, healthy fats are essential for the production of steroid hormones, while adequate protein intake supports the synthesis of growth and repair hormones. Aim for a well-rounded diet that includes all macronutrients in appropriate proportions.

2. Nutrient Timing: The timing of nutrient intake can also influence hormone levels. For instance, consuming carbohydrates before or after a workout can support insulin production and muscle glycogen replenishment. Additionally, including protein-rich foods in your meals and snacks throughout the day can help maintain stable blood sugar levels and support muscle protein synthesis.

3. Micronutrients: Micronutrients, including vitamins and minerals, are vital for optimal hormone function. For instance, vitamin D is necessary for the synthesis of hormones like testosterone, while zinc supports the production of thyroid hormones. Ensure you consume a diverse range of fruits, vegetables, whole grains, lean proteins, and healthy fats to obtain a broad spectrum of micronutrients necessary for hormone production and regulation.

4. Dietary Factors: Certain dietary factors can either positively or negatively affect hormone levels. For example:

- Fiber: Adequate fiber intake from whole foods, such as fruits, vegetables, and whole grains, can support healthy estrogen metabolism and balance.

- Sugar: High sugar consumption, especially from processed sources, can disrupt insulin function and lead to insulin resistance, affecting hormone regulation. It also decreases testosterone.

- Alcohol: Excessive alcohol intake can disrupt hormone balance, particularly impacting testosterone production and increasing estrogen levels.

- Caffeine: While moderate caffeine intake is generally safe, excessive consumption can elevate cortisol levels and disrupt sleep, which can impact hormone balance.

- Phytoestrogens: Certain plant compounds, like soy isoflavones, can exert mild estrogenic effects in the body, which may influence hormone levels. Their impact varies depending on individual factors and overall dietary balance.

5. Balanced and Varied Diet: Consuming a balanced and varied diet is essential for supporting optimal hormone function. Include a wide range of nutrient-dense foods, including lean proteins, whole grains, fruits, vegetables, nuts, and seeds. This approach ensures you obtain a diverse array of essential nutrients and phytochemicals that support overall health and hormone balance.

It's important to note that individual nutritional needs and hormone profiles may vary. Consulting with a registered dietitian or healthcare professional who specializes in hormone health can provide personalized guidance based on your specific needs and goals.

Exercise and Hormones

Different types of exercise can have distinct effects on hormone levels and metabolism. Here's an overview of how various training modalities can influence hormone production:

1. Resistance Training: Resistance training, such as weightlifting or bodyweight exercises, can have a significant impact on hormone levels. It stimulates the release of anabolic hormones, including testosterone and growth hormone, which are crucial for muscle growth and repair. Resistance training also improves insulin sensitivity, leading to better glucose metabolism and increased muscle glycogen storage.

2. Cardiovascular Exercise: Cardiovascular exercises, such as running, cycling, or swimming, can also influence hormone levels. It stimulates the release of endorphins, which are known as "feel-good" hormones that promote a sense of well-being. Regular cardiovascular exercise has been associated with improved insulin sensitivity, reduced levels of stress hormones like cortisol, and better regulation of appetite hormones such as ghrelin and leptin.

3. High-Intensity Interval Training (HIIT): HIIT involves short bursts of intense exercise alternated with brief recovery periods. This type of training can have a profound impact on hormone production and metabolism. It has been shown to increase growth hormone levels, improve insulin sensitivity, and enhance fat burning. HIIT also triggers the release of endorphins, leading to improved mood and motivation.

4. Other Training Modalities: Different exercise approaches, such as yoga, Pilates, and functional training, can also affect hormone levels. These modalities often incorporate elements of strength, flexibility,

and mindfulness. While they may not have the same direct impact on hormone production as resistance training or HIIT, they can contribute to overall well-being, stress reduction, and improved body awareness, which indirectly affects hormone balance.

Incorporating a variety of exercise modalities into your training program can provide synergistic benefits for hormone optimization. Combining resistance training to stimulate muscle growth and anabolic hormone release with cardiovascular exercise for cardiovascular health and stress reduction can lead to a well-rounded hormonal response. Additionally, integrating HIIT sessions to enhance metabolic function and fat burning can further support hormone balance.

It's important to note that individual responses to exercise may vary. Factors such as training intensity, duration, frequency, and individual fitness levels can influence the specific hormonal response. Consulting with a qualified fitness professional can help tailor an exercise program that aligns with your goals and optimizes hormonal benefits.

Stress Management

Stress management plays a crucial role in hormone optimization. Chronic stress can have a significant impact on hormone balance, leading to imbalances and related health issues. Here's why:

1. Cortisol Imbalance: Chronic stress triggers the release of cortisol, commonly known as the stress hormone. Prolonged elevation of cortisol levels can disrupt the balance of other hormones in the body. It can lead to reduced production of sex hormones like testosterone and estrogen, which can affect libido, muscle growth, and overall well-being.

2. Insulin Resistance: Chronic stress can also contribute to insulin resistance, a condition in which cells become less responsive to insulin. This can lead to imbalances in blood sugar levels, energy fluctuations, and increased risk of weight gain and metabolic disorders.

3. Thyroid Dysfunction: Stress can impact thyroid function, leading to imbalances in thyroid hormones such as T3 and T4. Thyroid hormones play a crucial role in metabolism, energy regulation, and overall hormonal balance. Disruptions in thyroid function can result in symptoms like fatigue, weight changes, and mood disturbances.

To manage stress and support hormone optimization, it's important to incorporate effective stress management strategies into your routine. Here are some strategies you can consider:

1. Relaxation Techniques: Engage in relaxation techniques like deep breathing exercises, progressive muscle relaxation, or guided imagery to promote relaxation and reduce stress levels. These techniques help activate the body's relaxation response, counteracting the effects of chronic stress.

2. Mindfulness and Meditation: Practice mindfulness and meditation to cultivate present-moment awareness and reduce stress. Regular mindfulness practice has been shown to lower cortisol levels, improve emotional well-being, and promote overall hormone balance.

3. Physical Activity: Regular exercise can be an effective stress management tool. Engaging in activities you enjoy, such as walking, jogging, yoga, or dancing, can help release endorphins, improve mood, and reduce stress levels.

4. Adequate Rest and Sleep: Prioritize quality sleep to support hormone regulation and stress reduction. Aim for consistent sleep patterns, create a relaxing bedtime routine, and ensure your sleep environment is comfortable and conducive to restful sleep.

5. Social Support: Cultivate a support network of friends, family, or community groups. Connecting with others and seeking support during stressful times can provide emotional relief and help manage stress more effectively.

6. Time Management and Prioritization: Practice effective time management and prioritize tasks to reduce stress and overwhelm. Break down large goals into manageable steps, delegate when possible, and establish boundaries to maintain a healthy work-life balance.

Managing stress is an ongoing process, and finding strategies that work for you is essential. Experiment with different techniques and prioritize self-care to minimize stress levels and optimize hormone balance. By proactively managing stress, you can support overall well-being and enhance the effectiveness of your hormone optimization efforts.

Hormone Testing & Monitoring

Hormone testing and monitoring play a crucial role in assessing hormone levels and identifying potential imbalances. Here's why it's important and an overview of different testing methods:

1. Assessing Hormone Levels: Hormone testing allows for a comprehensive assessment of hormone levels in the body. It provides valuable information about the functioning of various glands and the overall hormone balance. This information is essential for understanding the root causes of symptoms, optimizing health, and guiding appropriate interventions.

2. Identifying Imbalances: Hormone imbalances can lead to a range of symptoms and health issues. Testing helps identify specific imbalances, such as low testosterone, estrogen dominance, or thyroid dysfunction, which can guide targeted interventions and treatment plans.

3. Personalized Approach: Hormone testing provides an opportunity for a personalized approach to healthcare. It allows healthcare professionals to tailor interventions based on individual hormone profiles, considering factors such as age, sex, lifestyle, and specific health concerns.

Now, let's explore the different testing methods available:

1. Blood Tests: Blood tests are the most common method of hormone testing. They involve drawing blood samples and measuring hormone levels in the bloodstream. Blood tests provide a comprehensive view of hormone levels at a specific point in time and are particularly useful for assessing hormone levels that are tightly regulated, such as thyroid hormones or insulin.

2. Saliva Tests: Saliva tests measure hormone levels in saliva samples. Saliva testing is convenient, non-invasive, and can be done at home. It can assess the bioavailable (active) fraction of hormones and provide insights into hormone fluctuations throughout the day. Saliva testing is often used for assessing cortisol levels and hormone imbalances related to stress.

3. Urine Tests: Urine tests measure hormone metabolites excreted in the urine. This method offers insights into hormone metabolism and clearance. It can assess hormone levels over a more extended period, providing a broader perspective on hormone patterns. Urine tests are commonly used for assessing estrogen metabolites and hormone balance in conditions such as estrogen dominance.

Each testing method has its benefits and limitations:

- Blood tests provide a comprehensive overview of hormone levels but represent a snapshot of hormone status at a specific moment.

- Saliva tests offer insights into bioavailable hormone levels and diurnal hormone fluctuations but may not reflect overall hormone levels.

- Urine tests provide information about hormone metabolites and long-term hormone patterns but may not be as accurate for assessing hormone levels directly.

Interpreting hormone test results requires expertise and collaboration with a healthcare professional specializing in hormone optimization. They can evaluate the results, interpret them in the context of your symptoms and health history, and develop a tailored plan for hormone optimization.

Remember, hormone testing is just one part of the puzzle. It should be used in conjunction with a comprehensive assessment of symptoms, medical history, and lifestyle factors to guide effective interventions and optimize hormone balance. Working with a knowledgeable healthcare professional is essential for accurate interpretation and personalized treatment strategies.

Hormone Replacement Therapy (HRT)

Hormone replacement therapy (HRT) is a medical treatment option for individuals with clinically diagnosed hormone deficiencies or imbalances. It involves supplementing or replacing hormones that are not adequately produced by the body. Here's an overview of HRT, its types, benefits, and more:

1. Types of Hormone Replacement Therapy:

a. Bioidentical Hormones: Bioidentical hormones are synthesized to be structurally identical to the hormones naturally produced by the body. They are often derived from plant sources such as soy or yam. Bioidentical hormone therapy aims to restore hormone levels to their optimal range.

b. Synthetic Hormones: Synthetic hormones are chemically formulated hormones that are similar to those naturally produced by the body but not structurally identical. They are used in certain HRT approaches, such as oral contraceptives or traditional hormone replacement therapy.

2. Potential Benefits of Hormone Replacement Therapy:

a. Symptom Relief: HRT can alleviate symptoms associated with hormone deficiencies or imbalances, such as hot flashes, night sweats, mood swings, fatigue, and low libido.

b. Improved Quality of Life: By restoring hormone levels to a more optimal range, HRT can improve overall well-being, mood, energy levels, cognitive function, and sexual health.

c. Protection Against Certain Conditions: Depending on the hormone being replaced, HRT may offer protection against conditions such as osteoporosis, heart disease, and cognitive decline.

3. Importance of Professional Guidance:

a. Diagnosis and Assessment: Hormone deficiencies or imbalances require proper diagnosis and assessment by a healthcare professional. Through medical history review, symptom evaluation, and appropriate testing, they can determine if HRT is necessary and which hormones need to be addressed.

b. Personalized Treatment Plan: HRT should be tailored to individual needs. A healthcare professional will consider factors such as age, gender, medical history, current health status, and desired outcomes to develop a personalized treatment plan.

c. Monitoring and Adjustments: Regular monitoring of hormone levels and ongoing assessment of symptoms is crucial while undergoing HRT. Healthcare professionals can adjust dosages, treatment modalities, or medication types based on individual responses and changing needs.

d. Risks and Benefits Evaluation: HRT is not without risks. Working with a healthcare professional helps evaluate potential risks, side effects, and benefits based on individual circumstances, which may include factors such as age, medical history, and existing health conditions.

If you suspect a hormone imbalance or deficiency, it's essential to consult with a qualified healthcare professional who specializes in pediatric endocrinology. They will have the expertise to assess your condition and provide appropriate guidance and treatment options.

Hormone replacement therapy, such as testosterone replacement, is typically not recommended for adolescents unless there is a diagnosed medical condition that warrants such treatment. Hormone levels and development during adolescence are a natural and complex process, and it's important to allow your body to go through these changes naturally under the guidance of a healthcare professional.

If you have concerns about your hormone levels or development, it's important to have a comprehensive evaluation by a pediatric endocrinologist. They will conduct a thorough assessment, including medical history, physical examination, and appropriate laboratory testing, to determine if there is an underlying hormone imbalance or deficiency that requires treatment.

HRT is not suitable for everyone. It is typically recommended for individuals with clinically diagnosed hormone deficiencies or imbalances. The decision to pursue HRT should be made in consultation with a qualified healthcare professional who specializes in hormone optimization. They can assess your specific needs, discuss the potential risks and benefits, and guide you through the process of HRT, ensuring it aligns with your overall health goals and medical considerations.

Safety Considerations

When it comes to hormone optimization, it's crucial to prioritize safety and exercise caution. Hormones play a vital role in our overall health and well-being, and any interventions related to hormones should be approached with care and under proper medical guidance.

Hormone replacement therapy (HRT) and other hormone-related interventions should only be considered when there is a diagnosed medical condition or hormonal imbalance that requires treatment. It's important to work closely with qualified healthcare professionals, such as endocrinologists or hormone specialists, who have expertise in this field.

These professionals will conduct thorough evaluations, including comprehensive medical histories, physical examinations, and appropriate laboratory testing, to determine the need for hormonal interventions. They will also guide you through the potential risks, benefits, and alternatives associated with such treatments.

Hormone-related medications or supplements should not be self-prescribed or used without proper medical supervision. Hormones are powerful substances that can have significant effects on the body, and their misuse or inappropriate use can lead to adverse outcomes.

Additionally, it's important to be cautious when considering over-the-counter or online products that claim to boost or optimize hormones. Many of these products may lack scientific evidence or quality control, and their safety and efficacy cannot be guaranteed.

Ultimately, the importance of seeking proper medical guidance and supervision cannot be overstated. By working closely with qualified healthcare professionals, you can ensure that any interventions related to hormone optimization are done safely and responsibly, with your health and well-being as the top priority.

Individual Variations

Recognizing the individualized nature of hormone optimization is crucial when developing strategies for achieving hormonal balance and well-being. Every person is unique, and what works for one individual may not work the same way for another. Understanding and considering individual differences, genetics, and unique circumstances is key to developing effective hormone optimization strategies.

Hormone levels and responses can vary greatly among individuals due to factors such as genetics, age, lifestyle, and underlying health conditions. What may be an appropriate intervention for one person's hormone imbalance may not be suitable or necessary for another.

It's important to approach hormone optimization with an open mind and a willingness to explore different strategies and interventions. This may involve working closely with qualified healthcare professionals who can assess your individual needs, conduct appropriate testing, and develop personalized plans tailored to your specific circumstances.

Listening to your body and being attuned to its signals is also crucial. Pay attention to how your body responds to different interventions, whether it's changes in diet, exercise routines, stress management techniques, or other strategies aimed at optimizing hormone balance. What works well for you may not be the same as what works for someone else.

Additionally, it's important to be patient and persistent in the pursuit of hormone optimization. Achieving hormonal balance and well-being may require time, adjustments, and ongoing monitoring.

It's not a one-size-fits-all approach, and finding the right balance may involve trial and error.

The key is to approach hormone optimization with an individualized mindset, recognizing that what works for one person may not work for another. By considering your unique circumstances, genetics, and individual responses, and having a disciplined mindset, you can develop tailored strategies that support optimal hormone balance and overall well-being.

Additional Factors For Potential Testosterone Optimization

While some sources suggest that certain factors may have a minimal impact on testosterone levels, it's important to note that the scientific evidence supporting these specific strategies is limited, and their effects may vary among individuals. Here are a few additional points that have been mentioned in relation to potential testosterone optimization:

1. Minimize exposure to environmental estrogen-like compounds: Some studies suggest that certain chemicals found in plastics, pesticides, and other environmental pollutants may have estrogenic effects and potentially disrupt hormone balance. To minimize exposure, you can consider using glass or stainless steel containers for food and drinks, opting for organic products whenever possible, and being mindful of the products you use.

2. Competitive activities and challenges: Engaging in competitive activities, whether it's sports, games, or other challenges, has been associated with temporary increases in testosterone levels. These short-term increases are often attributed to the psychological and physiological responses to competition. However, it's important to note that these effects may be transient and may not have a significant impact on long-term testosterone levels.

3. Mindset and confidence: Some studies suggest that adopting a confident and assertive mindset may positively influence testosterone levels. Confidence-building activities, positive self-talk, and visualization techniques may help create a psychological state that supports optimal hormone balance. However, the impact of mindset on testosterone levels is complex and multifactorial, and individual responses may vary.

It's important to approach these additional strategies with caution, as their effects on testosterone levels may be minimal and highly individualized. It's also essential to prioritize overall health, well-being, and evidence-based approaches when considering hormone optimization. If you have concerns about your hormone levels or wish to explore ways to support optimal testosterone levels, consulting with a qualified healthcare professional would be advisable. They can provide personalized guidance based on your specific circumstances and help you make informed decisions.

XII: Injury Prevention & Management

Strategies for Preventing Common Injuries in Exercise

Engaging in regular exercise is crucial for maintaining a healthy and active lifestyle. However, it's important to prioritize injury prevention to ensure your fitness journey remains safe and sustainable. By implementing effective strategies, you can significantly reduce the risk of common injuries associated with resistance training and cardiovascular exercise. This guide will provide you with practical tips and techniques to help keep your workouts injury-free.

1. Proper Warm-up:

Begin each workout with a thorough warm-up routine to prepare your body for the demands of exercise. Incorporate dynamic stretches and movements that target the specific muscles and joints you'll be using. This increases blood flow, improves flexibility, and enhances muscle activation, reducing the risk of strains and sprains.

2. Correct Form and Technique:

Maintaining proper form and technique during exercise is paramount to prevent injuries. Focus on mastering the correct movement patterns and posture for each exercise. Start with lighter weights and gradually increase intensity as your form improves. Consider working with a qualified fitness professional or doing research on how to perform different exercises to ensure you're performing exercises correctly.

3. Gradual Progression:

Avoid the temptation to push yourself too hard or progress too quickly. Gradual and progressive overload is key to allowing your body to adapt and strengthen over time. Increase weights, repetitions, or intensity gradually to avoid overloading your muscles, joints, and connective tissues, which can lead to injuries.

4. Rest and Recovery:

Incorporate rest and recovery days into your training program. Rest is essential for allowing your body to repair and rebuild muscle tissue, reducing the risk of overuse injuries. Avoid training the same muscle groups on consecutive days and prioritize quality sleep to support optimal recovery.

5. Cross-Training:

Include variety in your exercise routine by incorporating cross-training. Engaging in different types of exercises and activities helps prevent overuse injuries by distributing the stress on your body more evenly. Cross-training also improves overall fitness, strength, and flexibility.

6. Listen to Your Body:

Pay attention to your body's signals and listen to any signs of pain, discomfort, or fatigue. Pushing through pain can lead to serious injuries. If you experience persistent pain or discomfort, modify or stop the exercise and seek professional advice if needed.

7. Proper Equipment and Gear:

Ensure you have appropriate equipment and gear for your chosen activities. Invest in well-fitting athletic shoes that provide proper support and cushioning. If you participate in high-impact activities, consider using supportive braces or protective gear to reduce the risk of joint and ligament injuries.

8. Balanced Muscle Development:

Focus on achieving balanced muscle development throughout your body. Imbalances in strength and flexibility between muscle groups can increase the risk of injury. Incorporate exercises that target all major muscle groups to maintain a balanced physique.

9. Injury Rehabilitation and Prehabilitation:

If you have a pre-existing injury or weakness, consult with a healthcare professional or physical therapist to develop a rehabilitation or prehabilitation program. This will help strengthen and stabilize the affected areas, reducing the risk of re-injury and promoting proper movement patterns.

10. Regular Assessments and Check-ups:

Schedule regular assessments and check-ups with healthcare professionals, such as physiotherapists or sports medicine specialists. They can evaluate your movement patterns, identify potential weaknesses or imbalances, and provide guidance on injury prevention strategies specific to your needs.

Incorporating these strategies into your exercise routine will help reduce the risk of common injuries related to resistance training and cardiovascular exercise. By prioritizing injury prevention, you can enjoy a safer and more sustainable fitness journey, allowing you to reach your goals while maintaining your physical well-being. Remember, injury prevention is a lifelong commitment, and by adopting these practices, you'll be on your way to a healthier and more enjoyable fitness experience.

Techniques For a Proper Warm-Up & Cool-Down

A well-executed warm-up and cool-down routine is essential for maximizing the benefits of exercise and reducing the risk of injury. The warm-up prepares your body for the upcoming physical activity, while the cool-down helps your body transition from exercise back to a resting state.

Warm-up Techniques:

1. General Cardiovascular Exercise:

Start your warm-up with light cardiovascular activities such as brisk walking, jogging, or cycling. This increases your heart rate, blood flow, and body temperature, priming your muscles for the upcoming workout.

2. Dynamic Stretching:

Incorporate dynamic stretching exercises that involve controlled, fluid movements through a full range of motion. Focus on major muscle groups and joints that will be involved in your workout. Examples include leg swings, arm circles, walking lunges, and torso rotations.

3. Joint Mobilization:

Perform exercises that gently mobilize your joints, promoting a better range of motion and joint stability. This can include shoulder rolls, ankle circles, wrist rotations, and neck movements. Move each joint through its full range of motion without forcing any painful or uncomfortable movements.

4. Sport-Specific Movements:

If you're engaging in a specific sport or activity, incorporate movements that mimic the actions and demands of that activity. For example, if you're about to play basketball, include light dribbling, shooting drills, or footwork exercises as part of your warm-up. If you're warming up for bench presses, perform a couple of bench pressing sets with lighter weights.

Cool-down Techniques:

1. Gradual Reduction of Intensity:

After completing your main workout, gradually reduce the intensity of your exercise. Slow down your pace or decrease the resistance on cardio machines. This allows your heart rate to gradually return to its resting state.

2. Static Stretching:

Include static stretching exercises during your cool-down. Focus on major muscle groups and hold each stretch for 15 to 30 seconds without bouncing. Stretching can help improve flexibility and reduce muscle soreness post-workout.

3. Foam Rolling or Self-Massage:

Use a foam roller or massage tools to target specific muscle groups and release any tension or tightness. This can help alleviate muscle soreness and promote recovery.

4. Deep Breathing and Relaxation:

Incorporate deep breathing exercises and relaxation techniques during your cool-down. This helps to reduce stress, promote a sense of calmness, and allow your body and mind to transition to a more relaxed state.

5. Hydration and Refueling:

Drink water to rehydrate your body after exercise. If your workout was intense or prolonged, consider consuming a post-workout snack or meal containing a balance of carbohydrates and protein to replenish energy stores and support muscle recovery.

Proper warm-up and cool-down techniques are essential components of any exercise routine. A well-executed warm-up prepares your body for physical activity, while a proper cool-down helps your body recover and return to a resting state. By incorporating these techniques into your workouts, you can enhance performance and reduce the risk of injury. Remember, dedicating a few extra minutes to warm up and cool down can make a significant difference in your exercise experience.

Rest & Recovery For Injury Prevention & Management

Rest and recovery are essential components of any successful training or exercise program. In the pursuit of our fitness goals, it's easy to overlook the importance of adequate rest and recovery, but neglecting these aspects can increase the risk of injuries and hinder progress. This guide highlights the significance of rest and recovery for injury prevention and management and provides strategies to incorporate them into your routine effectively.

1. Preventing Overuse Injuries:

Overuse injuries occur when the body is subjected to repetitive stress without sufficient time to recover. Rest days and proper recovery periods allow your body to repair damaged tissues, rebuild muscle fibers, and restore energy stores. By incorporating rest days into your training schedule, you reduce the risk of overuse injuries such as tendinitis, stress fractures, and muscle strains.

2. Muscle Repair and Growth:

During exercise, muscle fibers undergo micro-tears. Rest and recovery periods provide an opportunity for these fibers to repair and grow stronger. Without adequate recovery, muscles can become fatigued, leading to decreased performance and an increased risk of injury. Rest also allows the body to replenish glycogen stores and clear metabolic waste products, promoting optimal muscle function.

3. Balancing Hormones and Energy Systems:

Intense exercise places stress on the body's hormonal and energy systems. Rest and recovery help restore hormonal balance, especially the regulation of cortisol, a stress hormone that can impair recovery and increase the risk of injuries. Adequate rest also replenishes energy stores, such as ATP (adenosine triphosphate), allowing the body to perform at its best and reducing the risk of accidents caused by fatigue.

4. Managing Injuries and Rehabilitation:

In the event of an injury, proper rest and recovery become even more critical. Giving the injured area time to heal is crucial for effective rehabilitation. Depending on the severity of the injury, this may involve complete rest, modified activities, or specific rehabilitation exercises. Proper rest and recovery protocols, guided by healthcare professionals, can expedite healing, restore function, and prevent re-injury.

5. Strategies for Effective Rest and Recovery:

- Sleep: Prioritize quality sleep to promote physical and mental recovery. Aim for 7-9 hours of uninterrupted sleep each night.

- Active Recovery: Engage in light, low-impact activities such as walking, swimming, or yoga on rest days. This promotes blood flow, tissue repair, and helps reduce muscle soreness.

- Nutrition: Consume a well-balanced diet rich in lean proteins, healthy fats, and complex carbohydrates to provide the necessary nutrients for recovery and repair.

- Stress Management: Implement stress reduction techniques such as meditation, deep breathing exercises, or engaging in activities that promote relaxation. Chronic stress can impede recovery and increase the risk of injuries.

- Listen to Your Body: Pay attention to signs of fatigue, pain, or decreased performance. Adjust your training intensity, duration, or frequency accordingly to avoid overtraining and potential injuries.

Rest and recovery are integral parts of any training or exercise program. By prioritizing adequate rest, you allow your body to repair, rebuild, and adapt, reducing the risk of injuries and enhancing overall performance. Incorporate strategies for effective rest and recovery into your routine to optimize your training efforts, promote long-term health, and achieve your fitness goals safely. Remember, rest is not a sign of weakness but a crucial component of your journey toward optimal fitness and health.

Identify & Manage Common Injuries

Engaging in regular exercise and physical activity is essential for maintaining a healthy lifestyle. However, it's crucial to be aware of the potential risks of injuries that can occur during exercise. Muscle strains and joint pain are common injuries that can occur due to various factors, including improper form, overuse, or inadequate warm-up. This guide will help you identify and manage these common injuries effectively to support your fitness journey.

1. Muscle Strains:

Muscle strains occur when muscle fibers are overstretched or torn. They often result from sudden movements, improper technique, or inadequate warm-up. Common areas prone to strains include the hamstrings, quadriceps, calf muscles, and the muscles of the lower back.

Identification:

- Sudden pain or discomfort during exercise or movement

- Swelling, bruising, or tenderness in the affected area

- Limited range of motion and difficulty in performing certain movements

- Muscle weakness or inability to bear weight on the affected muscle

Management:

- Rest the injured muscle and avoid activities that worsen the pain.

- Apply ice packs or cold compresses to the affected area for 15-20 minutes every few hours during the first 48-72 hours to reduce swelling.

- Compress the injured muscle with a bandage or compression sleeve to minimize swelling and provide support.

- Elevate the injured limb if possible to reduce swelling.

- Use over-the-counter pain relievers, following the recommended dosage, to manage pain and inflammation.

- Gradually introduce gentle stretching and strengthening exercises as recommended by a healthcare professional or physical therapist.

- Seek medical attention if the pain is severe, persists, or if there is significant swelling or deformity.

2. Joint Pain:

Joint pain can occur as a result of repetitive stress, improper form, or underlying joint conditions such as arthritis. Common areas affected by joint pain include the knees, shoulders, hips, and wrists.

Identification:

- Pain, stiffness, or tenderness in the joint area during or after exercise

- Swelling, redness, or warmth around the joint

- Clicking or popping sounds during joint movement

- Limited range of motion or difficulty in performing certain exercises or activities

Management:

- Rest the affected joint and avoid activities that exacerbate the pain.

- Apply ice packs or cold compresses to the joint for 15-20 minutes every few hours during the first 48-72 hours to reduce swelling and inflammation.

- Support the joint with braces or wraps to provide stability and relieve stress.

- Use over-the-counter nonsteroidal anti-inflammatory drugs (NSAIDs) to alleviate pain and reduce inflammation, following the recommended dosage.

- Incorporate low-impact exercises and activities that do not put excessive strain on the affected joint.

- Seek professional advice from a healthcare provider or physical therapist for a proper diagnosis and personalized treatment plan, especially if the pain persists or worsens.

Being able to identify and manage common injuries related to exercise, such as muscle strains and joint pain, is crucial for maintaining your fitness journey safely. By recognizing the signs and symptoms of these injuries and implementing appropriate management strategies, you can aid in the recovery process and prevent further complications. Remember to prioritize proper form, warm-up adequately, and listen to your body to avoid injuries. If you experience persistent or severe pain, consult a healthcare professional for a thorough evaluation and guidance on the best course of action.

Seeking Medical Attention

While many exercise-related injuries can be managed through self-care and rehabilitation techniques, there are instances when it's crucial to seek medical attention. Knowing when to involve a healthcare professional and how to collaborate with them is vital for proper diagnosis, treatment, and effective recovery. This guide will provide insights into when to seek medical attention for an injury and offer strategies for working with healthcare professionals to facilitate your recovery process.

1. When to Seek Medical Attention:

It's important to recognize the signs that indicate a need for professional medical evaluation. Consider seeking medical attention in the following situations:

- Severe pain that persists or worsens despite self-care measures.

- Inability to bear weight on a limb or joint.

- Visible deformity or significant swelling around the injured area.

- Restricted range of motion or loss of function in a joint or muscle.

- Pain or discomfort accompanied by numbness, tingling, or weakness.

- Symptoms that interfere with daily activities or persist for an extended period.

2. Collaborating with Healthcare Professionals:

When seeking medical attention, it's essential to work collaboratively with healthcare professionals to ensure a proper diagnosis and develop an effective recovery plan. Here are some strategies for working with them:

- Choose the right healthcare provider: Depending on the nature of your injury, consult with an appropriate healthcare professional, such as a sports medicine physician, orthopedic specialist, or physical therapist, who specializes in musculoskeletal injuries.

- Provide a detailed history: Be prepared to provide information about the onset, duration, and specific symptoms of your injury. Mention any previous medical conditions or injuries that might be relevant.

- Participate actively in the evaluation: Engage in open and honest communication with your healthcare provider, describing your pain, limitations, and any activities that aggravate or alleviate the symptoms. This will aid in the accurate assessment of your condition.

- Ask questions: Seek clarification regarding your diagnosis, treatment options, and expected recovery timeline. Understand the purpose and potential side effects of prescribed medications or recommended interventions.

- Follow treatment recommendations: Adhere to the treatment plan prescribed by your healthcare provider, including medication, physical therapy exercises, or other interventions. Consistency and compliance are crucial for optimal recovery.

- Communicate progress and setbacks: Provide regular updates to your healthcare provider regarding your progress, including improvements, setbacks, or any new symptoms. This feedback will enable them to modify the treatment plan if necessary.

- Seek guidance for return to activity: Consult with your healthcare provider before resuming exercise or sports activities to ensure that you have fully recovered and can safely engage in physical activity again.

Knowing when to seek medical attention and how to work with healthcare professionals is essential for effective injury recovery. By recognizing the signs that indicate the need for professional evaluation and collaborating with experts in the field, you can receive appropriate diagnosis, treatment, and guidance tailored to your specific injury. Remember, the expertise and support of healthcare professionals play a significant role in optimizing your recovery process and helping you return to your active lifestyle safely.

XIII: Advanced Training Techniques & Terms

Overview of Advanced Training Techniques and Terms

In the realm of fitness and strength training, various training techniques are employed to stimulate muscle growth, enhance strength gains, and improve overall performance. Advanced training techniques, such as drop sets, supersets, and pyramid sets, can add variety, intensity, and new challenges to your workouts. This overview will provide insights into these advanced training techniques, their benefits, and how to incorporate them into your training regimen effectively.

1. Drop Sets:

Drop sets involve performing a set of an exercise to failure or near failure and then immediately reducing the weight and continuing with additional repetitions. This technique aims to extend the working set, intensify muscular fatigue, and target muscle fibers to a greater extent.

- How to perform drop sets: Start with a weight that allows you to perform a certain number of repetitions with proper form. Once you reach failure, reduce the weight by 10-20% and continue the exercise for additional repetitions. You can repeat this process with multiple weight drops if desired.

2. Supersets:

Supersets involve performing two different exercises back-to-back without rest. They can be performed for the same muscle group (e.g., targeting different heads of the biceps) or different muscle groups (e.g., alternating between chest and back exercises). Supersets increase training density and provide a time-efficient way to work multiple muscle groups.

- How to perform supersets: Choose two exercises that target the desired muscle groups. Perform one set of the first exercise, immediately followed by a set of the second exercise without resting in between. Rest for a short period after completing both exercises before starting the next superset.

3. Pyramid Sets:

Pyramid sets involve gradually increasing or decreasing the weight while decreasing or increasing the repetitions throughout a series of sets. This technique allows for progressive overload and challenges the muscles through different intensity ranges.

- How to perform pyramid sets: Start with a lighter weight and higher repetitions for the first set. Increase the weight while decreasing the repetitions for subsequent sets. Alternatively, you can start with heavier weights and lower repetitions and work your way up with lighter weights and higher repetitions.

Benefits of Advanced Training Techniques:

- Increased muscle fiber recruitment: Advanced techniques like drop sets, supersets, and pyramid sets challenge your muscles in unique ways, leading to increased recruitment of muscle fibers and potential for greater muscle growth.

- Enhanced muscular endurance: By pushing your muscles to fatigue with these techniques, you can improve their endurance capacity, allowing you to sustain performance during longer training sessions.

- Time-efficient workouts: Supersets and drop sets, in particular, can help you save time by combining exercises and reducing rest periods, making your workouts more efficient without compromising intensity.

Advanced training techniques like drop sets, supersets, and pyramid sets can add a new dimension to your workouts, stimulating muscle growth, improving strength gains, and enhancing overall performance. Incorporate these techniques strategically into your training program, gradually progressing in intensity, and paying attention to your body's response. As with any training method, it's important to prioritize proper form, listen to your body, and maintain a balanced approach to optimize your results and minimize the risk of injury.

Incorporating Advanced Training Techniques

Incorporating advanced training techniques like drop sets, supersets, and pyramid sets into your training program can bring variety, challenge, and potential benefits to your workouts. Here are some strategies to effectively implement these techniques:

1. Select the right exercises: Choose exercises that complement each other when performing supersets or drop sets. For example, pair a pushing exercise with a pulling exercise or target opposing muscle groups. For pyramid sets, select exercises that allow for incremental adjustments in weight and repetitions.

2. Plan your workouts: Determine which days or sessions you'll incorporate advanced techniques into your training program. You can assign specific exercises or muscle groups to each technique.

3. Progress gradually: Start with lighter weights and shorter sets when incorporating these techniques, especially if you're new to them. Gradually increase the intensity, weight, or number of sets as your body adapts and becomes more comfortable with the technique.

4. Focus on form and technique: Proper form is crucial for safety and effectiveness. Maintain proper technique throughout each repetition, even when performing high-intensity techniques. Avoid sacrificing form for the sake of adding more weight or repetitions.

5. Listen to your body: Pay attention to how your body responds to the advanced techniques. If you experience excessive muscle soreness, joint discomfort, or fatigue, adjust the intensity, volume, or

frequency of these techniques accordingly. Rest and recovery are essential for optimal progress and injury prevention.

6. Integrate progressive overload: Continuously challenge your muscles by gradually increasing the weight, repetitions, or intensity over time. This progressive overload principle ensures ongoing adaptation and growth.

7. Experiment and vary techniques: Don't be afraid to experiment with different variations of advanced techniques. For drop sets, try different weight reduction percentages or incorporate rest-pause techniques. With supersets, explore different exercise combinations and order. Varying the techniques can keep your workouts engaging and prevent plateaus.

8. Track your progress: Keep a training journal or use a fitness app to record your workouts. Note the weights used, sets, and repetitions for each exercise, including the advanced techniques. Tracking your progress allows you to monitor your performance and make informed adjustments to your training program.

9. Seek guidance if needed: If you're new to these advanced techniques or unsure about proper execution, consider working with a qualified fitness professional or strength coach. They can provide guidance, ensure the correct form, and tailor the techniques to your specific goals and abilities.

Remember, advanced training techniques should be used in moderation and within the context of your overall training program. They can be effective tools for adding intensity and variety, but they shouldn't replace the fundamentals of proper exercise selection, progressive overload, and balanced programming. Be patient, stay consistent, and enjoy the benefits these techniques can bring to your fitness journey.

Adjusting Your Training Program As You Progress

As you become more advanced and experienced in your training, it's important to adjust your program to continue making progress and challenging your body. Here are some key considerations and strategies for adjusting your training program:

1. Increase training frequency: As you become more advanced, you may benefit from increasing the frequency of your training sessions. This could involve adding an extra training day or splitting your workouts to focus on specific muscle groups more frequently.

2. Adjust volume and intensity: As your body adapts to your current training program, you'll likely need to increase the volume (number of sets and repetitions) and intensity (weight lifted) to continue stimulating muscle growth and strength gains. Gradually increase the weights you lift and the number of sets and repetitions you perform.

3. Incorporate advanced training techniques: Introduce advanced training techniques such as drop sets, supersets, pyramid sets, or rest-pause sets to add variety and challenge to your workouts. These techniques can help you break through plateaus and stimulate further muscle growth.

4. Focus on progressive overload: Progressive overload is the principle of gradually increasing the demands placed on your muscles to promote continuous adaptation. Look for opportunities to progressively increase the weights you lift, the number of sets and repetitions, or the intensity of your exercises.

5. Train different rep ranges: Vary your rep ranges to target different muscle fibers and stimulate muscle growth from different angles. Incorporate both lower rep ranges (1-5 reps) for strength and higher rep ranges (8-15 reps) for hypertrophy.

6. Prioritize compound movements: As you advance in your training, focus on compound movements that engage multiple muscle groups simultaneously, such as squats, deadlifts, bench presses, and pull-ups. These exercises provide a greater stimulus for overall strength and muscle development.

7. Optimize recovery: With increased training volume and intensity, proper recovery becomes even more crucial. Ensure you're getting adequate sleep, following proper nutrition, managing stress, and incorporating rest days into your training program. Listen to your body and make adjustments as needed to avoid overtraining.

8. Seek expert guidance if needed: If you're unsure about how to adjust your training program or want personalized guidance, consider working with a qualified strength coach or personal trainer. They can provide you with customized programming, technique feedback, and expert advice to help you reach your advanced training goals.

Consistency, patience, and gradual progression are key when adjusting your training program as you become more advanced. Always prioritize proper form, listen to your body, and make adjustments based on your individual needs and goals.

Common Fitness and Training Terms

Repetitions (Reps): The number of times you perform a specific exercise.

Sets: A group of repetitions performed consecutively with a brief rest period in between.

Rest Period: The time taken to recover between sets or exercises.

One Repetition Maximum (1RM): The maximum amount of weight you can lift for one repetition with proper form.

Progressive Overload: Gradually increasing the demands placed on the body during exercise to stimulate adaptation and progress.

Reps in Reserve (RIR): A method of gauging intensity where you stop a set when you have a specific number of reps left in the tank. For example, if you stop a set with 2 reps in reserve, it means you could have performed 2 more reps before reaching failure.

Rate of Perceived Exertion (RPE): A scale used to subjectively rate the intensity of an exercise or set. It typically ranges from 1 to 10, with 1 being very easy and 10 being maximum effort.

Superset: Performing two exercises back-to-back without resting in between. Usually, the two exercises target different muscle groups.

Drop Set: A technique where you perform a set of an exercise to failure, then immediately reduce the weight and continue the set without rest.

Pyramid Sets: Starting with a lighter weight and performing more repetitions, then gradually increasing the weight and decreasing the repetitions with each set.

Circuit Training: A form of exercise where you move from one exercise to another with minimal rest in between, targeting different muscle groups or performing different exercises in sequence.

Tempo: The speed at which you perform each phase of an exercise, including the concentric (lifting, shortening) and eccentric (lowering, lengthening) phases.

Volume: The total amount of work performed in a training session, typically calculated as sets x reps x weight.

Intensity: The level of effort or resistance used during an exercise.

Periodization: A systematic approach to organizing and varying training variables (such as volume, intensity, and frequency) over specific periods to optimize performance and prevent overtraining.

These are just a few of the many terms and concepts in fitness. Understanding these concepts can help you better navigate and plan your workouts.

XIV: Putting It All Together

Example Of a Workout & Nutrition Plan

Here's an example of a workout and nutrition plan for building muscle and losing fat. Please note that individual needs and preferences may vary, so it's always a good idea to consult with a fitness professional or nutritionist to tailor the plan to your specific goals and requirements.

Workout Plan:

Day 1: Push (Chest, Shoulders, Triceps)

Warm-up:

- 5-10 minutes of light cardio (e.g., brisk walking, cycling, or rowing)

- Barbell Bench Press: 3 warm-up sets

Workout:

1. Barbell Bench Press: 3 sets of 8-12 reps

2. Dumbbell Shoulder Press: 3 sets of 8-12 reps

3. Incline Dumbbell Fly: 3 sets of 10-15 reps

4. Tricep Dips: 3 sets of 10-15 reps

5. Cable Lateral Raises: 3 sets of 10-15 reps

6. Skull Crushers: 3 sets of 10-15 reps

Cool-down:

- 5-10 minutes of low-intensity cardio (e.g., walking or light cycling)

- Static stretches for the upper body (e.g., chest stretch, tricep stretch)

Day 2: Pull (Back, Biceps)

Warm-up:

- 5-10 minutes of light cardio (e.g., brisk walking, cycling, or rowing)

- Deadlifts: 3 warm-up sets

Workout:

1. Deadlifts: 3 sets of 8-12 reps

2. Lat Pulldowns: 3 sets of 8-12 reps

3. Barbell Rows: 3 sets of 8-12 reps

4. Hammer Curls: 3 sets of 10-15 reps

5. Seated Cable Rows: 3 sets of 10-15 reps

6. Preacher Curls: 3 sets of 10-15 reps

7. Barbell Shrugs: 3 sets of 8-15 reps

Cool-down:

- 5-10 minutes of low-intensity cardio (e.g., walking or light cycling)

- Static stretches for the upper body (e.g., back stretch, bicep stretch)

Day 3: Legs (Quadriceps, Hamstrings, Glutes, Calves)

Warm-up:

- 5-10 minutes of light cardio (e.g., brisk walking, cycling, or rowing)

- Walking Lunges: 3 sets of 10-15

Workout:

1. Squats: 3 sets of 8-12 reps

2. Leg Press: 3 sets of 8-12 reps

3. Romanian Deadlifts: 3 sets of 8-12 reps

4. Walking Lunges: 3 sets of 10-15 reps per leg

5. Leg Extensions: 3 sets of 10-15 reps

6. Standing Calf Raises: 3 sets of 12-15 reps

Cool-down:

- 5-10 minutes of low-intensity cardio (e.g., walking or light cycling)

- Static stretches for the lower body (e.g., hamstring stretch, quad stretch)

Day 4: Rest

Day 5: Push (Chest, Shoulders, Triceps)

Warm-up:

- 5-10 minutes of light cardio (e.g., brisk walking, cycling, or rowing)

- Incline Dumbbell Press: 3 warm-up sets

Workout:

1. Incline Dumbbell Press: 3 sets of 8-12 reps

2. Chest Press Machine: 3 sets of 8-12 reps

3. Dumbbell Chest Fly: 3 sets of 10-15 reps

4. Tricep Pushdowns: 3 sets of 10-15 reps

5. Lateral Raises: 3 sets of 10-15 reps

6. Skull Crushers: 3 sets of 10-15 reps

Cool-down:

- 5-10 minutes of low-intensity cardio (e.g., walking or light cycling)

- Static stretches for the upper body (e.g., chest stretch, tricep stretch)

Day 6: Pull (Back, Biceps)

Warm-up:

- 5-10 minutes of light cardio (e.g., brisk walking, cycling, or rowing)

- Dead Hangs or Banded Pull-Ups

Workout:

1. Pull-Ups: 3 sets of 8-12 reps

2. Seated Cable Row: 3 sets of 8-12 reps

3. Single-Arm Dumbbell Rows: 3 sets of 8-12 reps per arm

4. Hammer Curls: 3 sets of 10-15 reps

5. Cable Face Pulls: 3 sets of 10-15 reps

6. Concentration Curls: 3 sets of 10-15 reps

Cool-down:

- 5-10 minutes of low-intensity cardio (e.g. walking or light cycling)

- Static stretches for the upper body (e.g. back stretch, bicep stretch)

Day 7: Legs (Quadriceps, Hamstrings, Glutes, Calves)

Warm-up:

- 5-10 minutes of light cardio (e.g., brisk walking, cycling, or rowing)

- Smith Machine Squats: 3 warm-up sets

Workout:

1. Smith Machine Squats: 3 sets of 8-12 reps

2. Bulgarian Split Squats: 3 sets of 8-12 reps per leg

3. Romanian Deadlifts: 3 sets of 8-12 reps

4. Leg Extensions: 3 sets of 10-15 reps

5. Leg Curls: 3 sets of 10-15 reps

6. Seated Calf Raises: 3 sets of 12-15 reps

Cool-down:

- 5-10 minutes of low-intensity cardio (e.g., walking or light cycling)

- Static stretches for the lower body (e.g., hamstring stretch, quad stretch)

You can add some cardio at the end of your workouts or on rest days for extra calorie expenditure and overall health benefits.

Nutrition Plan:

- Consume a well-balanced diet that includes lean protein sources (e.g., chicken, fish, tofu), complex carbohydrates (e.g., brown rice, quinoa, sweet potatoes), healthy fats (e.g., avocados, nuts, olive oil), and plenty of fruits and vegetables.

- Aim for a calorie intake that supports your goals. To build muscle and lose fat, you may need to create a slight calorie deficit. However, ensure that you're still providing enough energy for your workouts and recovery.

- Prioritize protein intake to support muscle growth and repair. Aim for around 1 gram of protein per pound of body weight per day. Spread protein intake across all meals and snacks.

- Stay hydrated by drinking plenty of water throughout the day.

- Include pre-and post-workout meals or snacks to fuel your workouts and aid in recovery. These meals should contain a combination of protein and carbohydrates.

- Monitor your portion sizes and listen to your body's hunger and fullness cues. Practice mindful eating and avoid unnecessary snacking or emotional eating.

- Consider working with a registered dietitian or nutritionist to create a personalized nutrition plan based on your specific needs and goals.

Remember, consistency and adherence to both the workout and nutrition plans are key to achieving your desired results. It's essential to prioritize rest and recovery, listen to your body, and make adjustments as needed.

Adjusting Your Plan Based On Individual Preferences & Needs

Adjusting your workout and nutrition plan based on your individual needs and preferences is crucial for long-term success and sustainability. Here are some guidelines to help you make personalized adjustments:

1. Goals: Clearly define your goals, whether it's building muscle, losing fat, improving athletic performance, or maintaining overall health. Your goals will dictate the adjustments you need to make.

2. Training Frequency: Determine the number of days per week you can commit to training. If you have a busy schedule or prefer shorter workouts, you may opt for full-body workouts performed 3 times a week or upper/lower-body splits performed 4 times a week. If you have more time and prefer more specific training, you can increase training frequency to 4-6 days per week with different muscle group splits.

3. Exercise Selection: Customize your exercise selection based on your preferences and available equipment. If you enjoy free weights, focus on exercises like barbell squats and dumbbell bench presses. If you prefer bodyweight training, incorporate exercises like push-ups, lunges, and planks.

4. Intensity and Progression: Adjust the intensity of your workouts based on your fitness level and preferences. You can increase or decrease weights, adjust repetitions, or vary rest periods to challenge yourself appropriately. Gradually progress by adding weight, increasing repetitions, or performing more advanced variations of exercises as you get stronger.

5. Macronutrient Distribution: While maintaining a balanced diet, adjust your macronutrient distribution based on your specific goals and preferences. If you prefer a higher protein intake, increase protein-rich foods like lean meats, tofu, or legumes. If you feel more energized with higher carbohydrates, emphasize complex carbs like quinoa, whole grains, and fruits. Modify your fat intake based on your preferences for sources like avocados, nuts, or olive oil.

6. Meal Timing: Adjust meal timing based on your daily routine and personal preferences. Some individuals prefer three larger meals, while others prefer smaller, more frequent meals. Consider incorporating pre-and post-workout nutrition to optimize performance and recovery.

7. Listen to Your Body: Pay attention to how your body responds to the plan. If you experience excessive fatigue, muscle soreness, or lack of progress, consider adjusting the volume or intensity of your workouts or reevaluating your nutrition plan.

8. Seek Professional Guidance: If you're uncertain about how to adjust your plan or have specific needs or restrictions, consider working with a certified personal trainer or registered dietitian. They can provide expert guidance tailored to your individual requirements.

Remember, the key to successful adjustments is to be flexible and open to experimentation. It may take some trial and error to find the right balance that works for you. Continuously assess your progress, reassess your goals, and make necessary changes to keep your plan aligned with your individual needs and preferences.

Sustainability & Lifestyle Changes

Achieving long-term success in your fitness journey goes beyond short-term goals. It requires a shift in mindset and a focus on sustainability and lifestyle changes. Here's why sustainability is crucial and how to incorporate it into your approach:

1. Consistency: Consistency is key when it comes to reaching and maintaining your fitness goals. Crash diets and extreme workout regimens may deliver quick results, but they are often difficult to sustain over time. Focus on creating a plan that you can stick to consistently for the long run.

2. Balanced Approach: Embrace a balanced approach that encompasses both your physical and mental well-being. Don't restrict yourself too much or deprive yourself of the foods you enjoy. Instead, strive for moderation, portion control, and incorporating a wide variety of nutrient-dense foods into your diet. Similarly, find a workout routine that you genuinely enjoy and look forward to, rather than forcing yourself into activities you dislike.

3. Lifestyle Integration: Make fitness and healthy habits a part of your lifestyle, rather than viewing them as temporary measures. Integrate physical activity into your daily routine, whether it's taking the stairs instead of the elevator, going for a walk during breaks, or engaging in recreational activities you enjoy. Find healthy recipes and meal plans that suit your tastes and make them a regular part of your cooking repertoire.

4. Mindful Eating: Practice mindful eating by paying attention to your body's hunger and fullness cues. Eat slowly, savor each bite, and be present in the moment. Avoid distractions while eating, such

as watching TV or scrolling through your phone, as it can lead to mindless overeating.

5. Gradual Progression: Take a gradual approach to your fitness journey. Don't rush or push yourself too hard too soon, as it can lead to burnout or injury. Allow your body to adapt and progress at its own pace. Celebrate small victories along the way and acknowledge that progress takes time.

6. Flexibility: Be flexible and adaptable in your approach. Life is full of unexpected events and challenges that can disrupt your routine. Instead of getting discouraged, learn to adapt and find alternative ways to stay active and make healthy choices.

7. Self-Reflection: Regularly assess and reflect on your progress, challenges, and areas for improvement. Be honest with yourself about what is and isn't working. Adjust your strategies and goals accordingly, making necessary changes to ensure continued progress.

8. Support System: Surround yourself with a positive and supportive network of friends, family, or like-minded individuals who share your goals and values. Seek support when needed, whether it's through workout buddies, online communities, or professional guidance.

Remember, the ultimate goal is to create sustainable habits that become a natural part of your lifestyle. It's not about short-term perfection but rather long-term progress and overall well-being. By prioritizing sustainability and making gradual, realistic changes, you'll increase your chances of achieving and maintaining your desired results in the long run.

XV: Conclusion

Recap of The Key Lessons for Building Your Dream Body

1. Goal Setting: Set specific, measurable, achievable, relevant, and time-bound (SMART) goals to provide clarity and direction for your fitness journey.

2. Nutrition: Focus on a balanced and nutrient-dense diet that supports your goals. Prioritize whole foods, portion control, and macronutrient balance (protein, carbohydrates, and fats).

3. Exercise Routine: Design a well-rounded workout program that includes resistance training, cardiovascular exercise, and flexibility/mobility work. Incorporate progressive overload to challenge your muscles and promote growth.

4. Recovery and Rest: Understand the importance of rest and recovery in allowing your body to heal, adapt, and grow stronger. Ensure adequate sleep, manage stress, and include rest days in your training program.

5. Mindset: Cultivate a positive mindset, practice self-compassion, and focus on progress rather than perfection. Use affirmations and visualization techniques to stay motivated and overcome obstacles. Focus on developing self-discipline, so that even when you are going through hard times and aren't feeling motivated, you still do what's necessary.

6. Accountability and Support: Seek accountability through training partners, online communities, or professional guidance. Surround yourself with supportive individuals who share your goals and values.

7. Tracking Progress: Use various tools and strategies to track your progress, such as keeping a training journal, taking measurements, and regularly assessing your goals. Celebrate achievements and make adjustments as needed.

8. Self-Discipline: Build self-discipline and develop healthy habits by prioritizing consistency, overcoming excuses, and taking action even when motivation is lacking.

9. Injury Prevention: Prioritize proper warm-up and cool-down techniques, listen to your body, and gradually progress in your training program to prevent common injuries. Seek professional guidance if necessary.

10. Hormone Optimization: Understand the role of hormones in your body and how they influence various aspects of your fitness journey. Prioritize factors such as nutrition, stress management, and sleep for optimal hormone balance.

11. Sustainability: Emphasize sustainable lifestyle changes rather than quick fixes. Make fitness and healthy habits a part of your daily routine and focus on long-term progress and well-being.

Remember, building your dream body is a journey that requires dedication, patience, and consistency. Use these lessons and strategies as a foundation to create a personalized plan that aligns with your goals and values. Stay committed, stay focused, and enjoy the process of becoming the best version of yourself.

Commit to Your Goals and Embrace the Journey

Believe in Yourself: You possess the strength and determination to achieve your dreams. Embrace your abilities and have faith in your potential. Trust that you can overcome any obstacles that come your way. Every time you fail, you gain experience for the next attempt.

Start Today: Don't wait for the perfect moment. Begin taking small steps toward your goals right now. Every action you take, no matter how small, brings you closer to where you want to be.

Embrace the Process: Understand that transforming your body and life is a journey that takes time and discipline. Embrace the ups and downs, the victories and setbacks. Learn from challenges and use them as stepping stones to grow stronger.

Stay Consistent: Consistency is the key to progress. Commit yourself and your goals. Show up for yourself, day after day. Prioritize your workouts, nourish your body with healthy foods, and develop sustainable habits and lifestyle changes.

Embrace Challenges: Challenges are growth opportunities. Embrace them as learning experiences and opportunities for change. Overcome setbacks with resilience, determination, and a positive mindset.

Find Support: Surround yourself with positive, like-minded individuals who share your aspirations. Seek encouragement from friends, family, or fitness communities. Connect with those who uplift and motivate you.

Celebrate Milestones: Acknowledge and celebrate your achievements, no matter how small. Recognize the progress you've made and the efforts you've put in. Celebrate these moments to boost your confidence and keep your motivation strong.

Stay Focused on Your Why: Remind yourself of the reasons why you started this journey. Connect with the deeper meaning behind your goals. Let your why be your driving force when faced with challenges or moments of doubt.

Adapt and Adjust: Stay flexible and open to adjustments along the way. Your goals may evolve, and your needs may change. Embrace the opportunity to adapt your training, nutrition, and mindset to ensure continued growth and success.

Enjoy the Transformation: Embrace the transformation that occurs, not only physically but mentally and emotionally as well. Appreciate the positive changes that come with your journey. Embrace the process of becoming the best version of yourself.

Believe in your ability to achieve greatness. Take action, stay committed, and enjoy the journey toward your dream body and a fulfilling life. The power to create the life you desire lies within you. If you're reading this book, it's obvious that you are not settled for mediocrity and a normal lifestyle full of pleasure and regret, so get to work!

In Closing

Congratulations on reaching the end of this book! By now, you have gained valuable insights, practical strategies, and a wealth of knowledge to embark on your fitness journey with confidence and determination. You have learned that transforming your body and achieving your goals is not just a one-time endeavor but a lifelong commitment to your health and well-being.

Remember, your journey is unique to you. Embrace the process, stay consistent, and celebrate every milestone along the way. Understand that setbacks and challenges are a natural part of the journey, but they should never deter you from your ultimate vision. With the right mindset, perseverance, and a solid foundation of knowledge, you are well-equipped to navigate any obstacles that come your way.

As you move forward, keep in mind that this book is just the beginning of your ongoing education and growth. Stay curious, continue exploring new research, and remain open to evolving your approach as you gain more experience. Fitness is a journey of continuous learning and adaptation, and there is always more to discover.

Remember to listen to your body and prioritize self-care. Your body is an amazing machine, capable of incredible transformations, but it also needs rest, recovery, and nourishment. Take time to honor your body's needs, fuel it with nutritious foods, and prioritize quality sleep. Your commitment to overall well-being will contribute to long-term success and sustainable results.

Finally, never forget the power of your mindset. Believe in yourself and your ability to overcome challenges. Cultivate a positive inner dialogue, practice self-compassion, and surround yourself with a supportive community. Remember that your worth is not defined by your physical appearance but by the person you are and the positive impact you bring to the world.

Thank you for choosing this book as your guide on your fitness journey. It has been an honor and privilege to be a part of your transformation. Now, go forth and embrace the incredible potential within you. The power to build your dream body and live your best life is in your hands.

Wishing you strength, resilience, and unwavering determination as you create the body and life you truly deserve.

With utmost admiration and best wishes,

Bogdan Pashchynskiy

Don't miss out!

Visit the website below and you can sign up to receive emails whenever Bogdan Pashchynskiy publishes a new book. There's no charge and no obligation.

https://books2read.com/r/B-A-FGXY-IXGKC

BOOKS 2 READ

Connecting independent readers to independent writers.

About the Author

Welcome!

I'm Bogdan, embarking on a life-long journey of self-improvement. I firmly believe in the power of sharing knowledge and offering guidance to others, just as I would have wished for my younger self.

My utmost dedication lies in providing you with the most accurate and science-based information, coupled with actionable steps, to help you become the best version of yourself in the most efficient and effective way possible. My goal is to support you on your path, sparing you the trials and tribulations I've encountered along the way.

Whether you aspire to build strength, enhance your attractiveness, achieve weight loss, reach your goals, cultivate a resilient mindset, or expand your knowledge, you've arrived at the right destination.

Join me on this transformative journey as we dive deep into these captivating topics, exploring their nuances and discovering invaluable insights.

I sincerely hope that you find my books not only informative but also enjoyable companions on your quest for personal growth.

(For more of my work, including video content, my self-improvement journey, and science-based tips, feel free to check out my YouTube channel: 'Bogdan Pashchynskiy')

Best regards,

Bogdan

Read more at https://youtube.com/@Bogdan_PeakPerformance.

www.ingramcontent.com/pod-product-compliance
Lightning Source LLC
LaVergne TN
LVHW042346190726
843493LV00005B/931